Cognitive and Emotional Disturbance in the Elderly

Cognitive and Emotional Disturbance in the Elderly

CLINICAL ISSUES

Edited by

Carl Eisdorfer, Ph.D., M.D., & Robert O. Friedel, M.D.

Department of Psychiatry and Behavioral Sciences,
University of Washington, Seattle, Washington

YEAR BOOK MEDICAL PUBLISHERS, INC.

CHICAGO • LONDON

Printed in the United States of America.

Library of Congress Catalog Card Number: 77-77488

International Standard Book Number: 0-8151-3032-5

To Suzy and Sue, for reasons too many to elaborate here

Preface

TOYNBEE suggests in *Mankind and Mother Earth* that improvements in health and medical care leave man with a choice between early death or eventual senility. An awkward dilemma. This point of view, however, is shared by many and underlines the mixed blessing associated with increased life expectancy. The older group continues to be the fastest growing segment of our population. From 1960 to 1975 in the United States alone, that portion of the population over age 75 grew at a rate of about 36%. The implications of this significant increase among the elderly are vast. Currently there are over one million aged persons under long-term care and between 50% and 65% of them have significant problems of orientation, cognition, and emotion. The costs associated with caring for just this segment of the population are now in the range of $10 billion (fiscal 1976). As our population grows even older, the risks for cognitive and emotional problems are certain to increase and the cost of care will escalate accordingly.

As a result of the increase of older persons in our population, interest has shifted toward a more precise look at what is normal and abnormal in the functioning of the elderly. In keeping with this trend, the focus of this volume is on cognitive disturbance in the aged. The first section deals with a number of basic issues in age-related cognitive disorders, including recent studies in neuropathology, epidemiology, and in the role of stress. This is followed by articles on the evaluation of patients in and out of the institution from a medical as well as psychological perspective. The final section is devoted to treatment.

Treatment of patients with cognitive disabilities may be among the most broadly based in medicine because it involves the integration of good medical care and good nursing care within a supportive social environment which maximizes human potential while minimizing the need for professional supports. Decisions concerning whether or not to place patients in institutions are reflections on the role of social planning and the utilization of improved nutrition and/or medication. These issues are touched upon and, in some cases, developed by the contributors of this volume.

The primary purpose of this work is to make physicians in practice and other health care professionals aware of the rapidly emerging developments in the field of cognitive and related emotional disturbance in the elderly, particularly to alert them to the potential for reversibility of several syndromes which present as senile dementia, to raise the issue of viewing certain disorders as diseases rather than as naturally occurring consequences of old age, and to look broadly at the importance of the correct medical and social management of the aging patient.

Among the many issues which became apparent to the editors in putting together this volume, the most obvious was that of nomenclature. To the practicing clinician, terminology may seem trivial; yet it became clear to us that the different terms used to refer to the same or related conditions carry with them enormous differences in their implications for patient management. Thus, we discovered that the term *senile,* or *senility,* often used to describe this group of cognitive disorders, also indicated the expectation that deterioration was a normal and inevitable consequence of aging. If this were the case, we are then, of course, not dealing with a treatable illness, and palliative nursing care might be the best management strategy. Conversely, if we talk about Alzheimer's disease of late onset, we could view the disorder as a disease state with primary neuronal degeneration of unknown etiology. We would be interested in the most recent developments in the etiology of Alzheimer's disease and its treatment. Clearly, the disease connotes the possibility of prevention and/or treatment; therefore, patients suffering from a defined disease are much more likely to receive care, even when therapy is not currently available, just as patients with cancer are cared for in the hope that a new cure will be found.

Organic brain syndrome as a term to cover all difficulties which present a cognitive dysfunction also caused problems. The term may have some value if it is categorized as acute (reversible) or chronic (irreversible), both of which lend themselves to a variety of differential diagnoses. In the case of chronic organic brain syndrome associated with aging, the term *senile dementia* is most commonly used to identify one of three disorders of different etiologies, i.e., (1) senile dementia of the Alzheimer variant, (2) senile dementia of the cerebrovascular variant, or (3) senile dementia mixed. Since we have not established clearly their natural histories, it has been suggested that we do away with these diagnoses entirely. One suggestion found in Professor Isaac's chapter proposes the term *brain failure,* which would be analogous to renal or cardiac failure in that there are several potential etiologies for the condition and reversibility is certainly possible. Others have suggested the term *cognitive dysfunction* since it reflects what we observe in the patient rather than a diagnosis (of a disease) whose etiology is not clear, and the natural course of which is as yet moderately vague. *Dementia* alone as a diagnostic term was felt to be inadequate. Thus the decision was made that the term dementia not be used without such qualifiers as "cerebrovascular type," "Alzheimer type," or "mixed type"; where the origin is unclear, the use of the term *senile dementia* was permitted. *Senility,* wherever it was used alone, was discarded, as we hope it will be discarded from all professional diagnoses. We retained other individual usages, provided they were explained to the reader, in an effort not to infringe unduly on the prerogative of the contributors. Our main goal was to develop an internally consistent terminology.

Clearly, the terminology of cognitive disorders in later life needs systematic review with a focus on developing consistent usage. Currently we may find ourselves more confused than not. Just as improved nomenclature based on rigorous diagnostic criteria has done much in the last decade to improve the diagnosis and treatment of depressive disorders, so too will similar improvements in the field of cognitive disorders—particularly those found in later life—improve the diagnosis and treatment of those diseases. Finally, expanded efforts to define the etiologies of these disorders should lead to more enlightened, humane, and effective patient management. This volume should stimulate such efforts.

ACKNOWLEDGMENTS

In conjunction with the International Congress of Gerontology in Jerusalem, Israel, Sandoz Pharmaceuticals (U.S.A.) sponsored a workshop for physicians, psychologists, nurses, social workers, and other health care professionals who were concerned with problems of the aged. This Pre-congress Workshop was co-sponsored by the Israeli-Brookdale Institute on Aging and Adult Human Development in Jerusalem. In response to many requests for the publication of the papers and discussions presented at this workshop, the editors asked the participants to revise and update their material for publication in this volume. In addition, we have included edited versions of the valuable discussions of the Jerusalem conference, which, fortunately, had been tape-recorded.

We wish to thank Dr. Robert del Vecchio of Sandoz Pharmaceuticals for his support of the workshop and for his valuable personal contributions during and subsequent to the meetings, and Mrs. Deborah Green, our Editorial Associate, and Mrs. Mavis Graham for their help in the preparation of the final manuscript.

CARL EISDORFER
ROBERT O. FRIEDEL

Contributors

J. H. ABRAMSON
Head of Epidemiological Studies, Brookdale Institute of Gerontology and Adult Human Development; Professor of Social Medicine, The Hebrew University-Hadassah Medical School, Jerusalem, Israel

E. W. BUSSE, M.D., Sc.D.
Dean of Medical Education, Duke University Medical Center, Durham, North Carolina

WELTON R. CALVERT, M.S.W.
Program Specialist, Texas Research Institute of Mental Sciences, Houston, Texas

CARL EISDORFER, Ph.D., M.D.
Professor and Chairman, Department of Psychiatry and Behavioral Sciences, School of Medicine, University of Washington, Seattle, Washington

LEON EPSTEIN, M.D.
Professor of Psychiatry and Associate Director, Langley Porter Neuropsychiatric Institute, University of California, San Francisco, California

ROBERT O. FRIEDEL, M.D.
Associate Professor and Vice Chairman, Department of Psychiatry and Behavioral Sciences, School of Medicine, University of Washington, Seattle, Washington

CHARLES M. GAITZ, M.D.
Head, Special Clinical Services, Texas Research Institute of Mental Sciences, Houston, Texas

MIRIAM J. HIRSCHFELD, R.N., M.S.
Tel Aviv University, School of Continuing Medical Education, Department of Nursing; Kupat Holim, Dinah School of Nursing, Beilinson Medical Center, Tel Aviv, Israel

BERNARD ISAACS, M.D., F.R.C.P., M.R.C.P.
Charles Hayward Professor of Geriatric Medicine, University of Birmingham, Birmingham, England

ISRAEL KATZ, D.S.W.
Director, Brookdale Institute of Gerontology and Adult Human Development, American Joint Distribution Committee, Givat Ram, Jerusalem, Israel

DAVID W. K. KAY, M.D.
Professor of Psychiatry, The University of Tasmania, Hobart, Australia

HEINZ E. LEHMANN, M.D.

Director of Medical Education and Research, Douglas Hospital; Professor of Psychiatry, McGill University, Montreal, Quebec, Canada

LESLIE S. LIBOW, M.D.

Chief, Geriatric Medicine, Jewish Institute for Geriatric Care and Long Island Jewish-Hillside Medical Center, New Hyde Park, New York; Associate Professor of Medicine, Health Sciences Center, State University of New York at Stony Brook, New York

ITZCHAK MARGULEC, M.D., M.P.H.

Medical Director, American Joint Distribution Committee; Associate Director, Brookdale Institute of Gerontology and Adult Human Development; Visiting Professor in Social Medicine, The Hebrew University-Hadassah Medical School, Jerusalem, Israel

ROSEMARY McCASLIN, M.S.W.

Director, Senior Information Service, Texas Research Institute of Mental Sciences, Houston, Texas

JOYCE PARR SCHAIE, Ph.D.

Postdoctoral Fellow, Department of Psychology, University of California at Los Angeles, California

K. WARNER SCHAIE, Ph.D.

Director, Gerontology Research Institute, Ethel Percy Andrus Gerontology Center, University of Southern California, Los Angeles, California

ROBERT D. TERRY, M.D.

Chairman, Department of Pathology, Albert Einstein College of Medicine, Bronx, New York

HENRYK M. WIŚNIEWSKI, M.D., Ph.D.

New York State Institute for Basic Research in Mental Retardation, Staten Island, New York

Table of Contents

PART I

1 / Structural Aspects of Aging of the Brain

ROBERT D. TERRY, M.D.
Chairman, Department of Pathology, Albert Einstein College of Medicine, Bronx, New York

HENRYK M. WIŚNIEWSKI, M.D., PH.D.
New York State Institute for Basic Research in Mental Retardation, Staten Island, New York

THIS CHAPTER describes the results of studies designed to evaluate the relationship between organic changes in the brain and altered emotional and cognitive behaviors associated with the human aging process. An important finding resulting from these studies has been that we observe only quantitative, not qualitative, changes in brain structure in the brains of those with senile dementia as compared with those who have aged normally. One cannot help but wonder, then, whether we should consider that a pattern of continuous changes characterizes the passage from normalcy to that dreadful extreme, senile dementia.

In regard to the etiology of chronic organic brain syndrome in the elderly, or senile dementia, the popular concept for decades has been that it is due essentially to the effect of arteriosclerosis on the brain. Many neuropathologists have found that this is only occasionally the case, and statistics from the work of Tomlinson (1976) confirm this latter impression. Arteriosclerosis is clearly responsible for only about 20% of the cases of senile dementia. Most of these patients can be sharply demarcated by clinical history and by physical examination as having cerebrovascular disease rather than Alzheimer's dementia secondary to neuronal degeneration. Acute onset, stepwise course, and

NOTE: This work has been supported, in part, by grants from the National Institutes of Health, NS–02255, 03356, and 08180.

focal symptoms characterize the patient with vascular disease. An additional 12% of senile dementia cases are uncertainly related to arteriosclerosis. The vascular disease may take any of several forms: major ischemic lesions due to narrowing of carotid, anterior, or middle cerebral arteries; numerous microscopic infarcts in the cerebral cortex; or widespread subcortical ischemia as in Binswanger's disease. Hypertension may be an important factor in any of these varieties, and its treatment would undoubtedly lessen the frequency of senile dementia. Arteriosclerosis, however, is apparently not significantly involved in the great majority of cases of typical chronic organic brain syndrome in the aged.

The majority of cases, over 50%, are associated with changes in the brain, i.e., neurofibrillary tangles and neuritic (senile) plaques, which are essentially identical to those found in that presenile dementia which we call Alzheimer's disease. Many of us have therefore taken to using the same eponym, i.e., Alzheimer's dementia, for this common presenile dementia and for the most common form of dementia in the aged. In cases of primary neuronal degeneration, or Alzheimer's dementia, the brain displays a diffuse atrophy, usually most marked in the frontal and temporal regions. The arteries at the base of the brain are remarkably free of atherosclerosis and are widely patent. The blood flow has been found to be reduced in such cases. Nevertheless, most observers working in this physiological field now agree that the reduction in blood flow is secondary to the loss of cortical tissue with high metabolic needs. There is a poorly understood control system acting on the vessels of the brain, such that when parenchymal requirements are reduced, the blood flow is lowered. The parenchymal changes are not caused by the diminished blood flow; rather the reverse is true.

The cortical ribbon is narrowed, the white matter is shrunken, and the ventricles are somewhat enlarged. This atrophy of the brain is due to several changes, the best known of which is loss of neurons. Important studies by Brody (1955) twenty years ago quantified a dramatic neuronal loss most marked in the superior temporal cortex and to only a slightly lesser degree elsewhere in the cerebral cortex. He noted a decrease of almost 50% of cortical neurons in the so-called normal aged patients. This does not involve all areas of the brain, sparing at least some brain stem nuclei. In the very few counts which have been reported on older patients with chronic organic brain syndrome, there is a somewhat more severe loss, about 55–60% overall (Colon 1973). This counting, done by direct observation of tissue through a light microscope, is extraordinarily tedious. Recent computerized apparatus should make such counts more extensive and less time-consuming.[*] We really do not know why neurons are lost. A brain-reactive antibody has been found (Threatt et al. 1971) in the serum of aged humans and in certain old experimental animals. This may have something to do with lysis of neurons, but it is not yet proven, nor is it understood how such an antibody would pass what is apparently an intact blood brain barrier.

Another cause of cortical thinning is diminished extracellular space, i.e., the space between the cellular elements. This change has been demonstrated only in experimental animals and by the technique of freeze substitution, which is still somewhat disputed. Nevertheless, Bondareff (1973) has shown a drop from about 20% in the three-month-old rat brain to about 10% in the cerebral cortex and striatum of the aged rodent. This is associated, according to Bondareff, with a slowed spread of an exogenous transmitter substance injected into the brain parenchyma.

In the past few years some very exciting information has been made available (Mehraein et al. 1975 and Scheibel et al. 1975) concerning a diminished dendritic arborization found in both the aged human and the aged animal, at least of some species. Not only is there a lessened length of dendrites per neuron, but many dendrites have fewer spines. Since spines are the receptor portions of the synaptic complex, this loss would result in a marked physiological deafferentation and could cause profound functional change.

Neuropathologists have for several decades recognized two major microscopic changes in the aged brain: the neurofibrillary tangle of Alzheimer, and the senile or neuritic plaque. A very important prospective study by the group in Newcastle upon Tyne (Roth, Tomlinson, and Blessed 1966) demonstrated a strong correlation between the concentration of these lesions within the cortex and psychometric impairment. That is to say, the more impairment, the greater the concentration of plaques and tangles in the cortex. This does not prove a causal relationship between these lesions and the functional change, but it is highly suggestive of a strong and significant relationship.

The neurofibrillary tangle is to be found in the neuronal perikarya of the cerebral cortex, the amygdala, and, to a lesser extent, certain deeper structures. Through the light microscope, the lesion appears to

---

[*]Recent work (Terry et al. 1977) with computerized image analysis does not reveal differences between normal and demented patients in cell counts performed on samples of frontal or temporal cortex.

be an increased mass of argentophilic fibers irregularly traversing the neuronal cytoplasm. It must be emphasized, however, that small numbers of these abnormal aggregates are to be found in the normal aged; essentially all people beyond the age of 80, regardless of their mental state, have at least a few such lesions. It is a continuous spectrum of tissue change; in general, the more tissue change, the greater the mental impairment. The electron microscope (Kidd 1963; Terry, Gonatas, and Weiss 1964) reveals that the neurofibrillary tangle is made up of a bundle of submicroscopic fibers which partially displace the normal cytoplasmic organelles, leaving the nucleus structurally intact. At higher magnification, one sees that the individual fibers have a unique structure with periodic constrictions about every 800 Å, unlike any fiber to be found elsewhere in the human or in any animal tissue which we have so far examined. Our current understanding (Wiśniewski, Narang, and Terry, 1976) is that each of these remarkable fibers is about 220 Å in maximum width and appears to narrow every 800 Å to about 100 Å, and is made up of a pair of helically wound filaments, each of which measures about 100 Å. We have been particularly interested in the analysis of these fibers because they are structurally analogous to neurofilaments (100 Å) and neurotubules (240 Å) which are present in the normal nervous system of the human and other animals.

Chemical analysis of the whole brain tissue, however, fails in such situations to reveal any abnormality, probably because even though these structures are prominent through the microscope, they represent a relatively small portion of the tissue. However, by special methods (Iqbal and Tellez-Nagel 1972) one can isolate neurons in relatively pure bulk, and then analyze their subcellular contents.

In so doing, we find (Iqbal, Grundke-Iqbal, Wiśniewski, Korthals, and Terry 1976) three different sorts of significant fibrous proteins. First, microtubules which are normal structures within all cells, but especially prominent in neurons. They are straight tubules, and are made up of a protein dimer, the molecular weights of each monomer being 56,000 and 53,000 daltons. A second type of fibrous protein is the filament protein, the major electrophoretic component of which has a molecular weight of about 50,000 daltons. This seems to correspond to the 100 Å filament of normal neurons. A new protein, that which seems to represent the paired helical filaments, also has a molecular weight of about 50,000 daltons. Analysis of the peptides produced by tryptic digestion of each of these proteins indicates that among the normal filament protein, the twisted filament protein, and the smaller tubulin monomer, there is a very significant coincidence.

If this new protein from the abnormal, bifilar helix is truly new to the organism, then one must look for the mechanism by which a new protein can be produced in cells, i.e., by means of new genetic information. This could occur by means of genetic de-repression, i.e., activation of a gene which has been held dormant without expression in the cells. New genetic material could also be added by mutation, but this would not account for the great frequency. Or a slow virus might well be the means by which new genetic material gains access to the cellular mechanism, causing it to synthesize the abnormal new protein.

On the other hand, if it is found that this protein of the abnormal fibers is very similar to that which is normally present but has undergone some small modification to form the new twisted configuration, then we would consider different ways by which that could happen. Abnormal oxidation is a possibility, in which case, of course, one would be encouraged to treat these patients pharmacologically with antioxidants. Similarly, a misassembly of normal protein subunits might be responsible. In this regard, we must note that Crapper (1973) has demonstrated in senile dementia and in Alzheimer's presenile dementia a marked increase in the concentration of aluminum in the brain. This metal could perhaps be a de-repressor, or it might be the cause of misassembly. Aluminum has interesting experimental aspects in that it can, when injected into the subarachnoid space of certain susceptible animals, induce the formation of abnormal filamentous aggregates within neurons, related to, but significantly not identical to, those found in the human (Terry and Peña 1965).

The second major lesion to be found microscopically in the cerebral cortex is the neuritic or senile plaque which is located in the neuropil, measures 60–150 microns in diameter, and is made up of argentophilic rods and granules surrounding an amorphous core. Electron microscopy has proved what light microscopic staining techniques had indicated, i.e., that the central core is amyloid. The electron microscope showed that the rods and granules are actually neuronal extensions or neurites (Terry et al. 1964). Most of them are presynaptic terminals, and are abnormal because they contain twisted filaments (such as are found in the neurofibrillary tangles), laminated lysosomes, and degenerating mitochondria. Many synapses are involved, with the axonal side enlarged and containing abnormal organelles; the gap and dendritic side are unaltered. The amyloid core of the plaque is suggestive of an immunologic abnormality since at least some amyloid is said to be composed of fragments of gamma globulin light chains.

Of great interest is the recent evidence that in certain strains of susceptible mice a specific strain of scrapie agent can induce neuritic plaques almost identical to those of the human (Bruce and Fraser 1975). The scrapie agent is like a slow virus. It is found in nature in sheep and goats, but can be transmitted in cell-free filtrates to several other species. It ordinarily produces spongy changes in the brain which are very similar to those of a few diseases of humans which produce chronic organic brain syndrome: Creutzfeldt-Jakob disease and kuru, both of which are now known to be transmissible. The fact that neuritic plaques are found only with specific scrapie agents acting on specific strains of mice suggests the possibility that senile dementia might be the result of a widespread slow virus infecting genetically susceptible humans.

To summarize, we have reason to believe that senile dementia is related to loss of neurons, to diminished dendritic arborization, to loss of dendritic spines, to the tangles within the neuronal cell bodies, and to the numerous abnormal synapses within the neuritic plaques. The shrunken cerebral cortex is due to a loss of neurons, diminished arborization of the dendrites, and diminished extracellular space. The white matter shrinkage is due to a loss of the axons and their myelin following the death of the neuronal somata. The tangles are made up of the twisted filaments. The protein which comprises these abnormal structures has a molecular weight of about 50,000 daltons, and is closely related to normal neurofilaments and to normal microtubules. The neuritic plaques are made up of abnormal neurites containing bifilar helices, lysosomes, and degenerating mitochondria—the last two accounting, respectively, for the increased hydrolytic and oxidative activity of the plaques. Amyloid is present in the center of these plaques and gives rise to congophilia.

Although aging is seen as a set of complex psychological and sociological changes, these changes occur in a background of physical alterations of the nervous system, alterations that are measurable, visible, and undeniable. These physical alterations are, we believe, a significant part of the cause of senile dementia.

REFERENCES

Bondareff, W.: Age Changes in the Neuronal Microenvironment, in Rockstein, M. (ed.): *Development and Aging in the Nervous System* (New York: Academic Press, 1973).

Brody, H.: Organization of the cerebral cortex. III. A study of aging in the human cerebral cortex, J. Comp. Neurol. 102:511, 1955.

Bruce, M. E., and Fraser, H.: Amyloid plaques in the brains of mice infected with scrapie: Morphological variation and staining properties, Neuropathol. Appl. Neurobiol. 1:189, 1975.

Colon, E. J.: The cerebral cortex in presenile dementia. A quantitative analysis, Acta Neuropathol. (Berl.) 23:281, 1973.

Crapper, D. R., Krishnan, S. S., and Dalton, A. J.: Brain aluminum distribution in Alzheimer's disease and experimental neurofibrillary degeneration, Science 180:511, 1973.

Iqbal, K., Grundke-Iqbal, I., Wiśniewski, H. M., Korthals, J. K., and Terry, R. D.: Chemistry of Neurofibrous Protein in Aging, in Terry, R. D., and Gorshen, S. (eds.): *Aging, Vol. 3: Neurobiology of Aging* (New York: Raven Press, 1976), pp. 351–60.

Iqbal, K., and Tellez-Nagel, I.: Isolation of neurons and glial cells from normal and pathological human brains, Brain Res. 45:296, 1972.

Kidd, M.: Paired helical filaments in electron microscopy of Alzheimer's disease, Nature 197:192, 1963.

Mehraein, P., Yamada, M., and Tarnowska-Dzidusko, E.: Quantitative Study on Dendrites and Dendritic Spines in Alzheimer's Disease and Senile Dementia, in Kreutzberg, G. W. (ed.): *Advances in Neurology,* vol. 12 (New York: Raven Press, 1975).

Roth, M., Tomlinson, B. E., and Blessed, G.: Correlation between scores for dementia and counts of senile plaques in cerebral gray matter of elderly subjects, Nature 209:109, 1966.

Scheibel, M. E., Lindsay, R. D., Tomiyasu, U., and Scheibel, A. B.: Progressive dendritic changes in the aging human cortex, Exp. Neurol. 47:392, 1975.

Terry, R. D., Fitzgerald, C. A., Peck, A., Millner, J., and Farmer, P.: Cortical cell counts in senile dementia, Proc. Am. Assoc. Neuropathol., 1977. (In press)

Terry, R. D., Gonatas, N. K., and Weiss, M.: Ultrastructural studies in Alzheimer's presenile dementia, Am. J. Pathol. 44:269, 1964.

Terry, R. D., and Peña, C.: Experimental production of neurofibrillary degeneration. 2. Electron microscopy, phosphatase histochemistry and electron probe analysis, J. Neuropathol. Exp. Neurol. 24:200, 1965.

Threatt, J., Nancy, K., and Fritz, R.: Brain reactive antibodies in serum of old mice demonstrated by immunofluorescence, J. Geront. 26:316, 1971.

Tomlinson, B. E.: Personal communication, 1976.

Tomlinson, B. E., Blessed, G., and Roth, M.: Observations on the brains of demented old people, J. Neurol. Sci. 11:205, 1970.

Wiśniewski, H. M., Narang, H. K., and Terry, R. D.: Neurofibrillary tangles of paired helical filaments, J. Neurol. Sci. 2:173, 1976.

2 / The Epidemiology and Identification of Brain Deficit in the Elderly

DAVID W. K. KAY, M.D.
Professor of Psychiatry, The University of Tasmania, Hobart, Australia

THE EPIDEMIOLOGY of a disorder attempts to define its true prevalence and incidence in a population. Correct identification of those persons affected makes it possible to study their social, demographic, physical, and genetic characteristics. Cognitive impairment may result from many different pathological conditions, but in the brains of old people two types of changes, which may be called the senile and vascular degenerations, are by far the most common. Recent work (Corsellis 1962; Blessed, Tomlinson, and Roth 1968; Tomlinson, Blessed, and Roth 1970) has demonstrated a quantitative relationship between the presence and degree of impairment during life and the extent of the pathological changes at postmortem.

Before considering the problems of case identification, we may ask what is known of the epidemiology of brain deficit from the neuropathological point of view. It is the effects of such change which we are trying to identify during life.

Tomlinson (1972) studied the brains of an unselected group of patients of all ages coming to postmortem at a general hospital from any cause of death in the same way as he had earlier studied (Tomlinson, Blessed, and Roth 1970) the brains of elderly patients. He found senile plaques in the neocortex in 10–15% of those examined as early as the 4th decade, while the other types of senile change were first seen about a decade later. There was then a steep rise in the proportion of brains showing all these changes until, in the 10th decade, 70–80% showed senile plaques and granulovacuolar degeneration, and 100% showed Alzheimer's neurofibrillary tangles (Alzheimer's N.F.T.)

11

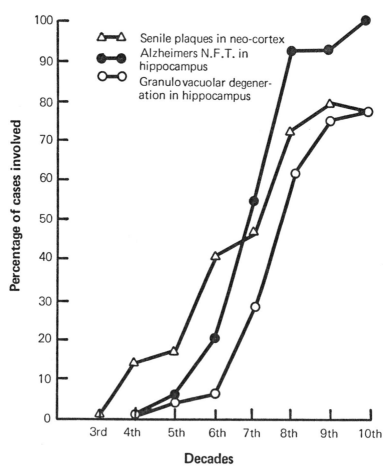

Fig 2–1.—Occurrence of senile plaques in the neocortex, and Alzheimer's neurofibrillary change and granulovacuolar degeneration in the hippocampus in 219 cases seen at autopsy (see Tomlinson 1972).

tangles in the hippocampus (Figure 2–1). This work bears out what Doctor Terry has been saying about the near-universality of pathological change with age, but it also suggests that the changes common in old age are the end product of processes that begin much earlier in life.

The shape of the curve in Figure 2–1, from Tomlinson's study of senile changes with age, shows a striking resemblance to the curve of first admissions to mental hospitals with "psychoses of the senium" (mainly organic psychoses) that is shown in Figure 2–2.

A variety of factors may affect admission rates, but there is also a

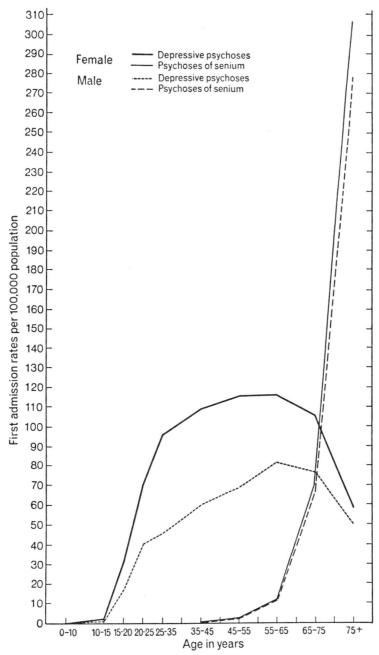

Fig 2–2.—Age and specific first admission rates to mental hospitals in England and Wales for 1966–67 for psychoses of the senium and affective disorders.

13

sharp increase with age in the prevalence of chronic brain syndrome (CBS) among people living at home (Table 2-1). The clinical-pathological changes shown to exist suggest that the resemblance of the curves is not fortuitous. In the 9th decade, the prevalence of chronic brain syndrome is at least 20%, and this figure would probably be considerably higher if all those very old people living in geriatric institutions were included.

In the Newcastle upon Tyne surveys, about an equal number of cases were thought to be due to vascular (chronic brain syndrome, arteriosclerotic type) as to senile dementia (chronic brain syndrome, senile type), and about 10-15% to other causes. However, this probably underestimates the real prevalence of senile change, because this change will seldom be diagnosed in the presence of localizing signs of brain damage, which, together with history of stroke, are the most important criteria for diagnosing vascular dementia. Neuropathological studies show that marked degrees of both types of change are found in the brains of about 20% of people with senile dementia.

In the elderly patients that Tomlinson studied (Blessed, Tomlinson, and Roth 1968; Tomlinson, Blessed, and Roth 1970), symptoms and behavior characteristic of senile dementia had been noted during life only in those who subsequently showed pathological changes of a certain degree of intensity. It was suggested that the threshold might be reached when plaque formation in the cortex corresponded to about 13 per field, or, in the case of vascular dementia, when the total volume of cerebral softening was 100 cc. The proportion of old people, in general, whose brains have these degrees of degenerative change is not known, however.

The differences between normal and abnormal aging appear, neuro-

TABLE 2-1.—PREVALENCE OF CHRONIC BRAIN SYNDROME°

		BOTH SEXES			MALES		FEMALES	
AGE	NO. TESTED	CBS	CBS %	SE	NO.	CBS %	NO.	CBS %
65-	253	6	2.4	± 0.9	110	3.6	143	1.4
70-	243	7	2.9	± 1.1	91	3.3	152	2.6
75-	144	8	5.6	± 1.9	51	5.9	93	5.4
80-	118	26	22.0	± 3.8	39	20.5	79	22.8
Total	758	47	6.2	± 0.9	291	6.2	467	6.2

Newcastle upon Tyne surveys among people aged 65 and over living at home.
CBS = chronic brain syndrome
SE = standard error of the percentage
°From Kay et al. 1970.

pathologically speaking, to be quantitative — not qualitative — but "case identification" means picking out individuals. An appropriate criterion in field studies is the point at which a person, through defects in memory, orientation, and grasp, can no longer carry on the activities of daily living. Lesser degrees of impairment may be strongly suspected, but the limits of normality are difficult to define precisely. Factors which may complicate identification of cases are the occurrence of focal lesions producing specific deficits, the presence of acute confusion, the effects of physical or emotional illness, the degree of domestic and social support, and the level of basic intelligence.

PREVALENCE OF CHRONIC BRAIN SYNDROMES

The rates reported from various parts of the world vary from 1.0 – 7.2% for "severe" dementia at ages 65 and over, with an addition of from 2.6 – 15% for "mild" dementia. "Mild dementia," however, is a nebulous concept and needs to be clearly defined before its prevalence can be investigated. Combined rates of 10 – 18% have been reported for "severe" plus "mild" dementia. I have suggested (Kay 1971) that the differences in reported prevalence rates are mainly due to differences in method and in criteria. When the method is a combination of inquiry with scrutiny of hospital records, the rates reported are low because presumably only the more disturbed, neglected, or socially impaired people are being identified. When representative samples of old people in the community are actually interviewed and their cognitive functions tested, the higher rates are reported.

It is generally agreed that chronic brain syndromes become progressively more frequent with advancing age. In the Newcastle upon Tyne surveys, which used the interview method, 20% of the old people aged 80 and over living at home were affected (see Table 2–1). Little is known, however, of the mental functioning of representative samples at extreme ages. After making allowance for age, the sexes are usually found to be equally affected. There is no conclusive evidence of a differential sex incidence of either senile or vascular changes in the brain.

METHODS OF CASE IDENTIFICATION

The method of interviewing elderly people in the field is the preferable method of identifying the prevalence of brain syndromes, and is the one on which the data reported in this article are based. In the Newcastle surveys the aim was to assess the nature and prevalence of psychiatric morbidity among representative samples of people aged 65 years or over living in their homes outside institutions, and to study its associations with medical and social variables. The method of selection was based on the Electoral Rolls in the manner described by Kay, Beamish, and Roth (1964). Interviewing was carried out on separate occasions by a psychiatrist and a social worker, and randomly selected subsamples were also tested by psychologists. (Savage et al. 1973). The results of follow-up were described by Kay et al. (1970) and by Bergmann et al. (1971).

When an old person is seen at home, answers should be sought to the following questions. Is there any evidence of failure or difficulty in carrying on the activities of everyday life? If so, can it be due to physical illness or disability, poor vision, or chaotic social conditions? If a cognitive factor seems probable, is this the result of recent brain damage or dysfunction, and not of something else, such as depression or mental subnormality?

In field surveys among randomly selected samples, the diagnosis of brain syndrome has to be based on relatively brief interviews and on investigations which are acceptable to the old person, and which are capable of being carried out in his home. The methods described here vary in the amount of expertise required. Apart from the intelligence tests, however, most of the tests described here could be adapted for use by nonmedical professionals.

1. Standardized intelligence tests. — Standardized intelligence tests and other special tests designed to measure psychomotor or perceptual functions, or new learning ability, are administered by psychologists. A separate interview is required. In our surveys it was possible to test 179 of 190 subjects on the Wechsler Adult Intelligence Scale (WAIS), but 30 of them were substitutes, matched for age and sex, for people who had recently died, refused to participate, or proved untestable. For the second part of the sample, a shortened form consisting of only the four subtests was used (vocabulary, comprehension, block design, and object assembly). The use of such tests gives valuable results, but they are difficult to use routinely for screening, since they involve much subject time and cooperation as well as special examiner skills. Also some old people cannot be tested because of severe motor or sensory disabilities, or because they are too mentally impaired to comprehend what is required.

2. Neurological examinations. — The neurological examination forms an essential part of the assessment of the medical status of an

old person, but in field studies only the presence of the major syndromes can be noted (e.g., hemiparesis, parkinsonism, pseudobulbar symptoms). This is within the scope of experienced nonmedical personnel. Cognitive impairment must be assessed independently of any neurological syndromes.

3. Tests of higher functions. — To test higher functions, the subject is asked to name simple objects, to point to named parts of the body, and to perform simple motor tasks (i.e., tests for aphasia, apraxia, left-right orientation). A full examination of the gnostic (higher order) functions will be outside the scope of the initial interview, but it is important to recognize the form of aphasia known as perseveration, which will alert the interviewer to the existence of organic deficit.

4. Scales for rating memory, orientation, and behavior. — Scales for rating memory, orientation, and behavior incorporate the simple questions, which are in general clinical use, for testing the sensorium and memory, or for eliciting descriptions of behavior. Unlike the ordinary clinical examination, the order in which the questions are asked and the method of scoring are standardized, and the total score gives a measure of overall performance. The Memory and Information Test (MIT) (Roth and Hopkins 1953) records current function only; an abbreviated and modified version of this test, shown in Table 2–2, was used in our surveys. The Dementia Rating Scale (DRS) (Blessed,

TABLE 2–2.—MEMORY AND
INFORMATION TEST*

QUESTION	SCORE, IF ANSWER CORRECT
How old are you?	1
When is your birthday? (month, date)	2
What year born?	1
What is today's date? (year, month)	2
(day of month, day of week)	2
Name two items of recent news?	2
Present monarch? (name and number)	2
Last monarch? (name and number)	2
Name of Prime Minister?	1
Name of last Prime Minister?	1
Date of Great War (First World War)?	2
(Year started, year ended)	
Date of Second World War?	2
(Year started, year ended)	
Maximum	20

*Modified from Roth and Hopkins, 1953.

Tomlinson, and Roth 1968) shown in Table 2–3, was also used. For the DRS an informant is asked specific questions about the subject's usual level of functioning during the past six months in the following areas: cognitive tasks and memory, habits, personality, and drives. Both these tests have been used as adjuncts to clinical assessment in our surveys, and not as the sole criteria for diagnosis. The MIT does not discriminate between acute and chronic brain syndromes, and to complete the DRS a reliable informant who is in regular contact with the subject has to be available. Originally, this scale was intended to measure cognitive impairment only, and the effects of purely physical disabilities were, so far as possible, excluded. Used in this way, with mostly ambulant mental-hospital patients, the scores have been found to correlate more highly than those on the MIT with the intensity of pathological changes in the cortex. This is presumably because the DRS attempts to measure persisting, and not merely transient, changes in mental state and behavior. In our domiciliary surveys, the DRS was used simply as a behavioral rating scale.

TABLE 2–3.—DEMENTIA RATING SCALE (SHORTENED FORM)*

CATEGORIES	SCORE PRESENT		ABSENT
Cognitive faculties and memory			
Inability to perform household tasks	1	½	0
Inability to cope with small sums of money	1	½	0
Inability to remember lists of three items (e.g., shopping)	1	½	0
Inability to find way about indoors	1	½	0
Inability to find way about familiar streets	1	½	0
Inability to grasp situations or explanations	1	½	0
Inability to recall recent events	1	½	0
Tendency to dwell in the past	1	½	0
Habits			
Eating: Cleanly, with proper utensils			0
Messily, with spoon only			1
Simple solids, e.g., biscuits			2
Has to be fed			3
Dressing: Unaided			0
Occasionally misplaced buttons, etc.			1
Wrong sequence, commonly forgetting items			2
Unable to dress			3
Excretion: Clean			0
Occasional accidents			1
Personal hygiene neglected:			
Frequent wet beds			2
Doubly incontinent			3

Instructions: The questions should be addressed to a reliable informant and refer to the patient's usual level of functioning over the past 6 months. Maximum score = 17.
*Modified from Blessed, Tomlinson, and Roth, 1968.

EXPERIENCE WITH RATING SCALES IN SURVEYS IN NEWCASTLE UPON TYNE

In the Newcastle studies we have had two aims. First, we wanted to identify those people showing symptoms of the kind and degree we were used to seeing in hospital patients with brain syndromes, to arrive at a prevalence rate for established cases. Second, we tried to record lesser degrees of impairment, comprising possible early, mild, or doubtful cases, which together might be placed under the umbrella term of "mild dementia." All the subjects were to be followed up (nearly all of them were), to confirm or refute the provisional diagnosis by reference to the later history, duration of survival, and cause of death. Unfortunately, the brains of only a very few of the subjects became available. Where the original diagnosis turned out in the follow-up to have been wrong, the case was reviewed and the sources of error examined. In this chapter, the data for organic syndromes refer to those subjects in whom the diagnosis was made or strongly suspected at initial interview and was not changed as a result of the follow-up 2½–3 years later.

Memory and Information Test.—The relationship of Memory and Information Test scores to clinical diagnoses are shown in Table 2–4. The raw scores were coded in groups for data processing: 0–5 (severely impaired); 6–10, 11–15, and 16–20 (good). The maximum score was 20 with this version of the test, as used in the domiciliary surveys (see Table 2–2). With a cutoff point between 10 and 11, discrimination is only fair, since 2% of the nonorganic cases, but 21% of the organic ones, are misclassified. If the cutoff point is 15–16, only 4% of the organic cases, but 20% of the nonorganic cases, are misclassified (the one organically ill subject who scored over 15 was suffering from myxedema). A cutoff point at 12–13 gave better discrimination in the subsample who were psychometrically tested,

TABLE 2–4.—MIT SCORES AND DIAGNOSIS°

PSYCHIATRIC DIAGNOSIS	SCORE						NO. TESTED	NOT TESTED
	0–10		11–15		16–20			
	NO.	%	NO.	%	NO.	%		
Normal	6	2	51	16	270	83	327	29
Functional	3	4	20	26	53	70	76	8
Senile dementia	18	78	4	17	1	4	23	4
Total	27	6	75	18	324	76	426	41

Newcastle upon Tyne survey among people aged 65 and over living at home.
°After Roth and Hopkins 1953.

TABLE 2-5.—DRS SCORES AND DIAGNOSIS*

PSYCHIATRIC DIAGNOSIS	SCORE						NO. TESTED	NOT TESTED
	≥ 10		5-9		0-4			
	NO.	%	NO.	%	NO.	%		
Normal	0	0	5	2	291	98	296	60
Functional	1	2	3	4	64	94	68	16
Senile dementia	5	23	11	50	6	27	22	5
Total	6	2	19	5	361	93	386	81

Newcastle upon Tyne survey among people aged 65 and over living at home.
*After Blessed, Tomlinson, and Roth 1968.

but this method has not yet been applied to the whole sample. Our data suggest that if this test were used as a screening device, further investigation of people scoring 12 or less would yield a high proportion of definite brain syndromes.

Dementia rating scale.—Results with the Dementia Rating Scale (Table 2-5) are less useful, principally because the DRS was not completed in 17% of the sample, usually because the old person was living alone or a reliable informant was not available at the time of the interview. The raw scores were coded as: 0-4 (normal); 5-9, 10 and over (severely impaired). Very few subjects scored over 7. Six—about 25%—of the individuals with senile dementia obtained scores in the "normal" range (0-4), but only nine (2.5%) of the nonorganic subjects scored more than 4. Review of the misclassified organic cases showed that they were a borderline group who caused diagnostic problems. Only one of them later deteriorated into a grossly demented state.

WAIS subtest scores and diagnosis.—Table 2-6 shows the tail of the distribution of scores. The lowest group of scores (≤6) was, with one exception, exclusive to subjects with senile dementia, but above this level there was considerable overlap. The WAIS scores, therefore, do not discriminate well, except at the lowest level—when the tests can hardly be done at all.

TABLE 2-6.—WAIS SUBTEST SCORES AND DIAGNOSIS

PSYCHIATRIC DIAGNOSIS	SUM OF SCORES ON 4 WAIS SUBTESTS					TOTAL
	≤ 6	7-12	13-18	19-24	≥ 25	
Senile dementia	6	3	2	2	0	13
Nonorganic	1	8	15	41	101	166
Total	7	11	17	43	101	179

Newcastle upon Tyne survey among people aged 65 and over living at home. Psychometrically tested subsample.

TABLE 2-7.—FOUR-YEAR MORTALITY AND MIT SCORES

| FOLLOW-UP | SCORE | | | | | | NO. TESTED | NOT TESTED |
| | 0-10 | | 11-15 | | 16-20 | | | |
	NO.	%	NO.	%	NO.	%		
Dead	15	20	12	16	49	64	76	10
Surviving	12	4	63	19	261	78	336	27
Not traced	0		0		14		14	4
Total	27	6	75	18	324	76	426	41

Newcastle upon Tyne survey among people aged 65 and over living at home.
Chi-square test: with 1 df (data divided at dotted line) χ^2 = 29.6, p < 0.001.

Validity of diagnosis.—While examination of the brains was seldom possible, clinical diagnosis was found to be very strongly associated with survival rates. Two thirds of the subjects with senile dementia had died at follow-up, compared with 16% of the remainder. The relationship between the MIT and the DRS scores and survival are shown in Tables 2-7 and 2-8. There are highly significant differences in mortality between subjects scoring within the "organic" and "normal" ranges on these tests.

Combination of tests.—The MIT and the DRS are intended to complement each other. When used together, and the cutoff points applied, 5% of organic cases were misclassified as nonorganic, and 8% of functionals and 1.4% of normals were misclassified as organic.

SOURCES OF ERROR IN CASE IDENTIFICATION

The main areas where assessment may be difficult and lead to diagnostic error appeared to be as follows:

1. Intelligence and Education

The value of the MIT for distinguishing subjects with low intelligence or poor education from those with brain syndromes is reduced

TABLE 2-8.—FOUR-YEAR MORTALITY AND DRS SCORES

| FOLLOW-UP | SCORE | | | | | | NO. TESTED | NOT TESTED |
| | ≥ 10 | | 5-9 | | 0-4 | | | |
	NO.	%	NO.	%	NO.	%		
Dead	5	7	12	16	56	77	73	13
Surviving	1	0	7	2	291	97	299	64
Not traced	0		0		14		14	4
Total	6	2	19	5	361	93	386	81

Newcastle upon Tyne Survey among people aged 65 and over living at home.
Chi-square test: with 1 df (data divided by dotted line) χ^2 = 39.6, p < 0.001.

by the questions about names and events, which very dull people may
not be able to answer. Such people are usually correctly orientated,
but the score on the DRS may be borderline, and diagnosis remain in
doubt. Several subjects in our survey, at first thought to be probably
"organic," were found not to have changed after 2–3 years, and were
reclassified as dull or subnormal. Of the people who were tested on
the WAIS, most of those with brain syndromes scored within the lowest 10%, but an equal number of nonorganic subjects obtained similar
scores. These nonorganic subjects seemed to represent the tail end of
the curve of the distribution of intelligence in the population. This
was shown in the following way. When organic and nonorganic subjects with low scores on the WAIS were compared for social class
(which was graded in five groups according to the Registrar-General's
method), the nonorganic cases were found to be of significantly lower
social class (p < 0.05). The crucial piece of information in interpreting
the scores is whether performance has markedly *deteriorated*—not the
actual level—and in a field survey the old person's former occupation
may be the only available clue.

2. Functional Psychiatric Disorder

Clinically, depression may simulate senile dementia, but the differences between the scores of the functionally ill and normal old people
on the tests, though significant, were not very striking. Of the four subjects with functional symptoms who scored in the organic range on the
DRS (see Table 2–5), two had already had strokes and one of these
deteriorated rapidly later. The third subject was stone-deaf, had bilat-
eral cataracts, and suffered from a paranoid psychosis. She was also
under treatment for myxedema. A diagnosis of brain syndrome might
have been justified in these three subjects. The fourth subject, a man
of 82, was moderately depressed, and his score on the DRS was probably incorrect.

Of the three subjects with functional illness who scored in the organic range on the MIT (see Table 2–4), one had been deaf from
childhood and could lip-read; unfortunately, she could not be followed up. Another was a woman of 80, who was at first thought to have
an early senile dementia, but was anxious and depressed. At follow-up
she had improved in all respects, and was rediagnosed as a high-grade
subnormal. The third was a depressed man of 73 who had hypertension and a hemiparesis from a recent stroke. He suffered another
stroke within a year.

We called such illnesses functional unless the scores on *both* tests were abnormal, or there were organic mental symptoms such as a perseveration, marked circumstantiality, or objective evidence of memory loss (purely subjective complaints of "bad memory" were usually a depressive symptom). This procedure means, of course, that our prevalence rates do not include all cases with known brain damage.

3. Impaired Hearing and Vision

The possible diagnostic problem of evaluating patients with sensory deficits was addressed. In our study, subjects with severe loss of hearing or sight did not usually cause difficulty in diagnosis unless there was another condition present. Thus, a woman of 90, who was very deaf and had cataracts in both eyes, also had chronic rheumatoid arthritis which prevented her from feeding or dressing herself and from carrying out household tasks. Her rating within the organic range on the DRS was probably mainly due to these latter disabilities, but she also scored just within the organic range on the MIT. Brain syndrome was not diagnosed, however, because she was alert and in touch, and not disorientated.

4. Acute or Chronic Physical Illness

We encountered very few people who happened to be going through an episode of acute confusion associated with physical illness, no doubt because these states are usually transient and end either in death, or else, in the absence of an underlying chronic syndrome, in complete recovery.

Chronic physical disability may cause difficulty in scoring on the DRS. However, in our experience, there are relatively few old people in unselected domiciliary samples whose physical disabilities are so severe that they obtain scores within the range of senile dementia cases on tests like the MIT and DRS. It is different with patients in geriatric medical wards. The MIT is useful for assessing present cognitive function even in severely physically ill patients.

RECENT STUDIES

Shapiro et al. (1956) showed that many of the time-honored clinical tests of the sensorium (such as the "cowboy story," serial sevens, digits forward and backward), as well as certain intelligence tests, failed to differentiate patients with and without brain damage when precautions were taken to avoid "contamination" of clinical diagnosis by the results on the very tests whose validity was being studied. With the recent increase in interest in the epidemiology of mental deterioration in the elderly, efforts have been made to improve the measuring instruments. This usually involves removing items found to be redundant, because they are too easy or too difficult; experimenting with methods of scoring; attempting to increase reliability between clinicians by careful definition of items and standardization of procedures; and by making sure that the tests adequately sample different aspects of cognitive function.

Shortened form of the Memory and Information Test. – Hodkinson (1972) showed that the original long form of the MIT could be shortened to ten questions without losing much information, and proving more convenient and acceptable. The ten questions are: age, time (to nearest hour), address for recall at end of test, year, name of hospital, recognition of two persons, date of birth, year of First World War, name of present monarch, counting backward (20 – 1). This test was recommended as suitable for assessing the elderly in institutional care. It closely resembles the version used in the Newcastle study (see Table 2 – 2).

Dementia rating test. – The original DRS test was shortened (see Table 2 – 3) by omitting the items concerned with "personality" and "drives" which were found to be measuring something different from the other questions and which were also probably the least reliable items.

Psychogeriatric Assessment Schedule. – The Psychogeriatric Assessment Schedule is being developed by Klaus Bergmann and colleagues in Newcastle (Bergmann et al. [in press]). The aim is to produce a reliable method of screening to be employed by nonmedical members of the primary care team in assessing organic and functional syndromes in old people on the lists of general practitioners. The diagnoses produced are at present being validated against the judgment of an experienced psychiatrist who is interviewing the same people. The design is based on a "decision-making model," combined with an experimental approach, which will eventually determine the weights to be given to each item and the cutoff points to maximize the differentiation between diagnostic groups. In Module 1 the subjects are assessed for social competence and self-care. Those found to be incompetent are first assessed to see if physical disability is involved (Module 2) before being tested for organic symptomatology (Module 3), while the remainder pass straight to Modules 4 and 5, where they are assessed for functional symptoms. Social competence and self-care is measured by ability to do the shopping and housecare, and to carry out personal toilet, and on the degree of mobility and need for nursing or other help in the home. Recognition of organic symptoms is based on (1) behavior and appearance; (2) ability to communicate; and (3) a fourteen-question test of orientation for place, time, and persons.

Geriatric Mental State Schedule.—The Geriatric Mental State Schedule has been developed by Copeland and his associates (Copeland et al. [in press]) with the aim of improving reliability of psychiatric diagnosis and the rating of psychiatric symptoms in geriatric subjects. The Schedule is based on items from the Present State Examination (PSE) and Psychiatric Status Schedule (PSS), but there are modifications to make it easier for interviewing elderly subjects, and a number of new sections for assessment of cognitive function have been added. A method of scoring is used which takes note of the degree of error, and whether the subject is aware that he does not know the answer. There are also sections dealing with body and object recognition (the face/hand test), naming of objects, perseveration, forced grasping, and delusions. Apart from the behavior items, reliability of the Schedule is satisfactory. A shortened form, suitable for use for screening, has also been developed.

CONCLUSION

Some of the methods which have been used for the identification of brain syndromes in field surveys among the elderly have been described, and some of the sources of difficulty or error discussed. Screening techniques and interviewing schedules are being developed which should improve the reliability of diagnosis, and may have the effect of increasing further the correlations between the presence of chronic brain syndrome and criterion variables, such as the rate of mortality and the degree of pathological change in the brain when examined after death. These advances should prove of value both in planning services for the older portion of the population, and for anticipating the probable future needs of individual elderly patients and their families.

ACKNOWLEDGMENTS

Dr. Klaus Bergmann was responsible for the interviewing and clinical tests, and Dr. R. D. Savage and Dr. Peter Britton, for administering the WAIS. Miss Eleanor Foster assisted with the data processing. The surveys in Newcastle upon Tyne were supported by a grant from the

Department of Health and Social Security, which was administered by Professor Sir Martin Roth and the University of Newcastle upon Tyne.

REFERENCES

Bergmann, K., Gaber, L. B., and Foster, E. M.: The development of an instrument for early ascertainment of psychiatric disorder in elderly community residents: A pilot study. (In press.)

Bergmann, K., Kay, D. W. K., Foster, E. M., McKechnie, A. A., and Roth, M.: A Follow-up Study of Randomly Selected Community Residents to Assess the Effects of Chronic Brain Syndrome and Cerebrovascular Disease, in *Psychiatry*, Part II: Excerpta Medica International Congress Series no. 274 (Amsterdam: Excerpta Medica, 1971).

Blessed, G., Tomlinson, B. E., and Roth, M.: The association between quantitative measures of dementia and of senile change in the cerebral grey matter of elderly subjects, Br. J. Psychiatry 114:797, 1968.

Copeland, J. R. M., Kelleher, M. J. Kellett, J. M., Gourlay, A. J., Gurland, B. J., Fleiss, J. L., and Sharpe, L.: The Geriatric Mental State Schedule—development and reliability, Psychol. Med. (In press.)

Corsellis, J. A. N.: *Mental Illness and the Ageing Brain* (London: Oxford University Press, 1962).

Hodkinson, H. M.: Evaluation of a mental test score for assessment of mental impairment in the elderly, Age Ageing 1:233, 1972.

Kay, D. W. K., Bergmann, K., Foster, E. M., McKechnie, A. A., and Roth, M.: Mental illness and hospital usage in the elderly: A random sample followed up, Compr. Psychiatry 11:26, 1970.

Kay, D. W. K.: Epidemiological Aspects of Organic Brain Disease in the Aged, in Gaitz, C. M.(ed.): *Ageing and the Brain* (New York: Plenum Press, 1971), pp. 15–27.

Roth, M., and Hopkins, B.: Psychological test performance in patients over 60. Senile psychosis and affective disorders of old age, J. Ment. Sci. 99:439, 1953.

Savage, R. D., Britton, P. G., Bolton, N., and Hall, E. H.: *Intellectual Functioning in the Aged* (London: Methuen, 1973).

Shapiro, M. B., Post, F., Löfving, B., and Inglis, J.: "Memory function" in psychiatric patients over sixty, some methodological and diagnostic implications, J. Ment. Sci. 102:233, 1956.

Tomlinson, B. E.: Morphological Brain Changes in Non-demented Old People, in van Praag, H. M., and Kalverboer, A. F. (eds.): *Ageing of the Central Nervous System* (Haarlem: De Erven F. Bohn, N. V., 1972), pp. 38–57.

Tomlinson, B. E., Blessed, G., and Roth, M.: Observations on the brains of demented old people, J. Neurol. Sci. 11:205, 1970.

3 / Stress, Disease and Cognitive Change in the Aged

CARL EISDORFER, PH.D., M.D.
Professor and Chairman, Department of Psychiatry and Behavioral Sciences, School of Medicine, University of Washington, Seattle, Washington

IN MANY THEORIES OF AGING, the concepts of stress and disease have been acknowledged as critical elements in hypotheses concerning physical and mental dysfunction. Stress is presumed to accelerate aging processes. However, it may specifically mediate vulnerability to physical disease, as well as facilitate previously initiated age-related physiological degeneration. Stress may compromise ability to respond or impair the reserve capacity of the organism. Alternatively, stress may be a challenge-yielding, improved, long-term adaptation. This chapter identifies key theoretical and research issues relevant to an improved understanding of stress in the etiology and pathogenesis of changes observed with advancing age.

DEFINITIONS AND METHODOLOGICAL ISSUES

The introduction of stress as a systematic explanatory construct in the life sciences is credited to Hans Selye. His seminal contributions (1936, 1946, 1950, 1970, and 1976) describing the reactive physiologic state, the general adaptation syndrome which prepares the individual for "flight or fight" have had a major influence on researchers in the behavioral and biological sciences. The term stress remains ambiguous, however, and with increasing usage has become less precise. For the engineer, stress refers to an external force directed at some physical object, and strain is the result of this force, causing temporary alterations in the structure of the object (Lazarus 1966). Unfortunately, behavioral scientists have defined the term less consistently, and many seemingly diverse lines of inquiry (i.e., anxiety, disasters, frustration, conflict, psychosomatic disorders, disease and other factors)

27

have been investigated under the rubric of "stress" research (Appley and Trumbull 1967).

For the most part, studies on stress have involved little cross-disciplinary cooperation and have been defined narrowly within biological, psychological, or sociological paradigms. This has only amplified the multitude of definitions, with the result that stress has remained a diffuse construct (Levine and Scotch 1970), often criticized as "unscientific" and useless.

Stress is presumed to occur in reaction to stimuli — physical, psychological, or social. Stressful stimuli have been characterized as being "intense," "rapidly changing," "unexpected," as well as productive of boredom or frustration (Appley and Trumbull 1967). In general, stressors have been regarded as either unpleasant or overwhelming to the adaptive capacity of the organism. The perception and appraisal of stress is a function of stimuli characteristics as well as individual factors such as previous experience, ability, personality, environmental constraints, health, and education (Appley 1967; Lazarus 1966; Lazarus et al. 1974).

Responses to stress can be grouped into three categories: (1) physiological responses; (2) behavioral responses, including expressions of affect; and (3) subjective states, self-reported (Moss 1973). Both Lang (1968) and Lazarus (1968) have discussed these three parameters for the measurement of stress responses in detail, citing evidence justifying a threefold classification. Although useful, methodological confusion has resulted since the three are not well correlated, as will be discussed. According to Selye (1956), the physiological response to stress involves three temporal phases: (1) the alarm reaction; (2) the stage of resistance involving an increased capacity of the organism to respond; and (3) exhaustion, characterized by a loss of functional capacity. Physiological responses indicative of the stress response include modification of heart rate, respiration, vasomotor and galvanic skin responses, as well as changes in endocrine activity. One complex factor in evaluating biobehavioral responsivity to stress is the problem of individual variation. The intercorrelation between various measures of physiological reactivity (heart rate variability, electrodermal response, plasma-free fatty acids, blood pressure, and finger blood volume) is not high (Wilkie 1976). This physiological reaction has prompted observers from as long ago as Galen to Dunbar (1935) to a host of contemporary investigators (Engel 1962; Lowenthal and Chiriboga 1973; Groen 1975; Selye 1950, 1976; Eisdorfer and Wilkie 1977; Woolf 1975; Wittkower and Dudek 1975) to link stress with disease both as a cause and as an effect.

In brief, behavioral responses include erratic performance, mal-coordination, increased errors, fatigue, and perseverative behaviors, as well as tremors, stuttering, somatic symptoms, and depressive affect (Paykel et al. 1967). Subjective verbal responses indicate anxiety or tension and include reports of somatic symptomatology, and depression.

A rather broad array of situations is presumed to induce stress. These include rapid cultural change, work, examinations, battle conditions, concentration-camp confinement, impending surgery, and illnesses. The underlying assumption of numerous studies investigating the relationships among life events and susceptibility to illness is that life changes require adaptation and are stressful, depending on the severity of the change. Life crises such as loss of a loved one, or job demotion (Mechanic 1968), as well as retirement, children leaving home (Lowenthal 1974; Carp 1972), or relocation (Lawton and Nahemow 1973), have been investigated, as has the hypothesis that an accumulation of life changes occurring within a limited period of time may be related to the development of an illness (Rahe and Lind 1971; Rahe and Paasikivi 1971; Dekker and Webb 1974; Edwards 1971; Holmes 1970; Rahe 1968; Wyler, Masuda, and Holmes 1971).

Many presumably routine situations are also reported to be stress-inducing. Experienced auto drivers have exhibited cardiovascular changes and even angina when driving in city traffic. Accountants show marked elevations in serum cholesterol levels and blood clotting times during the tax-filing period (Friedman et al. 1958).

In overview, a number of issues emerge in interpreting stress-related research. First, since there are individual differences in perception, few situations will be perceived by all individuals as stressful and, indeed, a situation that is stressful to an individual one time may not be stressful at another (Appley and Trumbull 1967). Such variables as age, personality, intellectual ability, health (expressed genetically, physiologically, or subjectively) may affect the subject's perception of the situation as well as his coping style (Janis 1974; Lazarus et al. 1974). Second, relatively little attention has been paid to the sequence and predictability of stress-inducing events. It is often difficult to determine whether an event precedes the stress or the reaction precedes the event. This is a major methodological problem in studies of retirement (Carp 1972) or "empty nest" transitions (Harkins 1974). Third, a frequent, albeit erroneous, assumption is that stressful events always lead to impaired performance. The data indicate that moderate stress may improve functioning (Broadbent 1971; Broverman et al. 1974; Eisdorfer 1968; Ellis 1975). Fourth, investigators often err by measuring one variable, such as galvanic skin response (GSR), heart rate (HR), or blood pressure (BP), and assuming that other measures will vary simultaneously. This may not be the case (Lacey 1967; Bridges 1968; Wilkie 1976).

Fifth, the multiplicity of approaches and definitions in studies of stress predictably leads to a certain amount of confusion. Although the confusion may be reduced within a given discipline, the utility of narrow, reductionistic studies is questionable. Stress reactions involve multiple, simultaneous physiological, subjective, and behavioral reactions.

A primary methodological focus for the future should be a clarification of the specificity, selectivity, and patterning of multiple, concurrent responses to stress, emphasizing the sensitivity of the organism to psychosocial parameters (Mason 1971, 1975). A significant body of data suggests that the "nonspecific" stress response postulated by Selye (1950) is erroneous (Mason et al. 1968; Mason 1971, 1975). Individuals are capable of responding to a range of physical and behavioral stimuli with a wide variety of complex and synergistic responses. The compelling task for the biobehavioral scientist is to determine the biobehavioral mechanisms which mediate either a pathological or adaptive response, and to determine the differential vulnerability of the individual to stressful stimuli throughout the life span.

BIOBEHAVIORAL CONCOMITANTS OF STRESS

Although the neuroendocrine system behaves as a functional organizational unit, subsystems may be analyzed separately. One subsystem, the sympathetic-adrenal medullary system, stimulates catecholamine secretion in response to psychosocial factors (Mason 1972). There is, however, relatively little information on age-related changes in catecholamine metabolism among humans. This is unfortunate since catecholamine release is a primary stress response and catecholamines seem to respond to a wider spectrum of stressor stimuli than other homones (Mason 1975). Karki (1956) noted increased resting urinary excretion of catecholamines from ages 1 to 50 years with a slight but consistent decrease between ages 60 and 90 years. However, Frolkis (1966) has postulated that decreasing levels of these circulating neurotransmitters leads to increased sensitivity of the aged to the catecholamines.

Eisdorfer and colleagues (Eisdorfer, 1973) report more pronounced free fatty acid (FFA) mobilization in the peripheral circulation (a direct correlation with catecholamine levels) among aged men (60–80 years) than among young men (25–45 years) during verbal learning. They proposed that deficits in performance among the aged may be associated with heightened autonomic nervous system receptor activity in specific target organs. Although supporting data have been reported (Eisdorfer et al. 1970; Herr and Birren 1973), the generality of these interpretations is still subject to question (Froehling 1974; Eisdorfer, Nowlin, and Wilkie [in ms.]), and further work is still needed to investigate the heightened sensitivity to autonomic arousal in the aged.

If, indeed, older persons show heightened autonomic reactivity to certain stimuli or events and/or if older individuals over-attend to, or misinterpret, signals originating from such autonomic activity, the result would be an increased sensitivity to somatic events, as in hypochondriasis. At higher levels of stress, almost all persons would experience such signals as unpleasant. Studies in the perception of autonomic state differences (including biofeedback control of autonomic state) would be quite valuable in shedding more light on the relationship between internal receptors of physiologic state and behavior. The hypothesis that response inhibition, or cautiousness, in older persons is secondary to the psychophysiologic effects of stress consequent to perceived failure is well worth exploration.

Stress occurs not only in response to environmental situations, but also as a consequence of particular personality variables and possible genetic factors. These sets of factors are related, since personality structure and genetic traits may also influence life situation. As Levi (1971) suggests, however, while it is well established that physical environmental stimuli can cause many diseases, the role that psychosocial stimuli play in disease causation is not clear. One notion is that stress is a nonspecific physiologic response of the body, related to the rate of wear and tear in the organism, and consequently to an increased morbidity and mortality associated with a variety of diseases (Levi and Kagan 1971). It has been suggested that however valuable the physiologic reactions to stress may have been in mobilizing behavior such as fighting or escaping in the early history of mankind, they have ceased to be universally appropriate as a basis for dealing with the more subtle socioeconomic and psychological conflicts of a modern and typically urban society. In most instances today socialization patterns necessitate control of emotions and aggressive motor activities. This creates the potential for discordance between the socialized expression of emotion, the neuroendocrine concomitants of emotion, and the psychomotor impulses likely to accompany the physiological state. If it lasts long enough, this conflict may be of pathogenic significance (Levi, 1974). Since the older organism is presumed to be less able to cope with such challenges (Marx, 1974; Timaris, 1972), it would appear appropriate to clarify the relationship of conflict and stress in the etiology of pathology with advancing age.

As methodological improvements have resulted in more refined research designs, clinical opinions about anxiety and neuroticism have been replaced by sophisticated psychological measures. Among these have been the Minnesota Multiphasic Personality Inventory (MMPI) and the Cattell 16 Personality Factor Inventory (16PF) (Jenkins 1971). It is important to note that many studies using such tools have supported the hypothesis that middle-aged as well as older men who develop coronary disease are more anxious.

Rosenman and Friedman have described a behavior pattern (type A) which has been associated with coronary disease among middle-aged men. Type A is defined as a style of living characterized by excesses of competitiveness, time urgency, restlessness, acceleration of common activities (e.g., walking, eating), hostility, hyperalertness, and explosiveness of speech amplitude — but not manifest anxiety. It is of interest to note that type A behavior alone is a poor predictor of cardiovascular disease (CVD) among the aged (Rosenman et al. 1964, 1966), and those past age 59 were eliminated from the data analysis of the 8½ year follow-up study (Rosenman et al. 1970). Since the relationship between type A behavior and CVD was based upon the initial evaluation of behavior (Rosenman and Friedman 1971), it would be valuable to know whether this behavior type is modified with increasing age. Rosenman (1974) has postulated that if the challenges or conflicts of the milieu were removed, the type A behavior pattern might change. Although most of the research in this area has been limited to men, type A women have similar outcomes and indeed show biochemical changes similar to those noted in high-risk men (Friedman and Rosenman 1957; Kenigsberg et al. 1974). Investigation into the mechanisms and intervention techniques is obviously desirable.

LIFE EVENT CHANGES

Although genetic parameters are important determinants in understanding vulnerability to disease throughout the life span, life events are also critical variables to consider in the onset of illness. Based upon the assumption that major changes in life are stressful, with effects which may be cumulative over limited periods, thereby affecting susceptibility to disease, Holmes and Rahe developed the Schedule of Recent Experience (SRE) over many years to estimate the impact of life changes on the onset of illness. A scaling instrument, the Social Readjustment Scale (Table 3–1), was also developed to assess the amount of life change in each of the SRE events (Holmes and Rahe 1967). The SRE consists of 43 items of varying consequence and attributed weight, positive as well as negative. They range from minor traffic violations and job promotions to death of spouse. A significant accumulation of life-change units increases susceptibility to disease (Holmes and Holmes 1970; Holmes and Masuda 1973; Rahe 1974; Rahe and Arthur 1968). Individuals whose lives are in a relatively steady state of psychosocial adjustment, on the other hand, tend to report little illness (Rahe 1969). The higher the score, the greater the likelihood of developing a wide variety of illnesses — infections, accidents, metabolic dysfunction, myocardial infarcts, and minor health problems. Rahe (1974, p. 58) also states that ". . . constitutional endowment helps to explain an individual's susceptibility to particular types of illness, but does little to explain why an individual develops an illness at a particular point in time . . . ."

The SRE assumes that life change is stressful regardless of the event experienced. Whereas the SRE work is impressive, the logic of combining positive and negative events is questionable (Brown 1974; Mechanic 1975; Sarason, DeMonchaux, and Hunt 1975). Vinokur and Selzer (1975) have published data using an adaptation of the SRE which provided separate ratings for positive and negative life events, as well as measures related to depression, stress, anxiety, paranoia, and aggression. Only negative life events were systematically related to the dependent variables measured.

Future research designed to build on the valuable reports in the literature using the SRE should include evaluation of individual differences and self-ratings of positive or negative impact of events, as well as events relevant to populations varying by age and culture.

The relationship between accumulated changes in life events and health among the aged is a critical one which has not been extensively studied. The developmental context in which changes may occur is important. Life changes should be evaluated to determine the extent to which the individual has control over the event, previous experience in dealing with such changes, resources for coping, health status, and degree of anticipation and preparation (Lowenthal and Chiriboga 1973; Nelson 1974; Sarason and Johnson 1976). Since the

TABLE 3-1.—THE SOCIAL READJUSTMENT
RATING SCALE*

LIFE EVENT	MEAN VALUE
1. Death of spouse	100
2. Divorce	73
3. Marital separation	65
4. Jail term	63
5. Death of close family member	63
6. Personal injury or illness	53
7. Marriage	50
8. Fired at work	47
9. Marital reconciliation	45
10. Retirement	45
11. Change in health of family member	44
12. Pregnancy	40
13. Sex difficulties	39
14. Gain of new family member	39
15. Business readjustment	39
16. Change in financial state	38
17. Death of close friend	37
18. Change to different line of work	36
19. Change in number of arguments with spouse	35
20. Mortgage over $10,000	31
21. Foreclosure of mortgage or loan	30
22. Change in responsibilities at work	29
23. Son or daughter leaving home	29
24. Trouble with in-laws	29
25. Outstanding personal achievement	28
26. Wife begin or stop work	26
27. Begin or end school	26
28. Change in living conditions	25
29. Revision of personal habits	24
30. Trouble with boss	23
31. Change in work hours or conditions	20
32. Change in residence	20
33. Change in schools	20
34. Change in recreation	19
35. Change in church activities	19
36. Change in social activities	18
37. Mortgage or loan less than $10,000	17
38. Change in sleeping habits	16
39. Change in number of family get-togethers	15
40. Change in eating habits	15
41. Vacation	13
42. Christmas	12
43. Minor violations of the law	11

*From Holmes, T. H. and Rahe, R. H.: The social readjustment rating scale, J. Psychosom. Res. 11:213, 1967. Used by permission of Pergamon Press Ltd. See this article for complete wording of the items.

number of life changes (at least as our tools measure them) apparently decreases with increasing age (Holmes and Holmes 1970; Lowenthal 1974), one should be able to detect whether fewer changes would be required to affect health status in old age—particularly if the system is already weakened by disease—or whether the slower rate of change protects the more vulnerable aged.

LIFE SPAN ANALYSIS OF STRESS AND LIFE CHANGES

Neugarten (1970) suggests that life events may not constitute as severe a stress if they occur in an appropriate time of life. Thus, although the death of a spouse is usually a traumatic event, the aged are more prepared for such losses by experience with peers and may have a less severe reaction than the young. Data indicate that widows over 65 fare better than anticipated (Heyman and Gianturco 1973), depending upon financial circumstances (Atchley 1975), although widowers may do less well (Parks et al. 1969; Gerber et al. 1975).

Predictably, areas of concern differ at different ages and according to sex, as indicated in a recent study by Lowenthal and colleagues (1975). For young newlyweds, a major concern is anticipation of parenthood; for the postparental age group, the men are concerned with work-related problems, while the women tend to be more concerned with children and their own personal growth.

Whereas good health and no crises were the dominant themes for preretirement men, the impact of impending retirement concerned women at this same age (Lowenthal 1975). The number of life changes decreased from the newlywed stage to the postparental stage and remained fairly stable through the imminent retirement stage.

It is not clear whether major life-style transitions such as retirement or children leaving home (i.e., "empty nest") are universally stressful. Neugarten (1970) and Lowenthal and Chiriboga (1972) found no association between the "empty nest" state and emotional well-being. This was supported by Harkins (1974); however, she also obtained indices of physical health and observed that women going through this period had more physical problems than women in the pre-or-post "empty nest" periods. As noted by Harkins (1974), much of the earlier research failed to include individuals at all stages of the transition.

Studies frequently fail to control for such variables as experience, preparedness, and resources available. Changes over time are highlighted by Stokes and Maddox (1967) who observed that blue-collar workers were more satisfied with retirement than white-collar workers initially, but after three to five years become dissatisfied while the white-collar workers remain unchanged. There is a need for research spanning the temporal stages of a transition before any conclusion can be reached about the relationship between stress and its possible pathological consequences.

AGE INTERACTION WITH DEPENDENT VARIABLES

Many of the dependent variables used in stress research, such as impaired behavioral performance or physical and emotional problems, occur with increasing age independent of apparent stress. In physiological studies involving young animals, prolonged stress may produce signs of premature aging, such as loss of hair, wrinkling of skin (Selye 1970). In the older organism, the pathology secondary to stress may be impossible to differentiate from changes relating to age and/or preexisting disease. While deviant emotional states are a frequent measure of stress in the young, depression, for example, may increase generally with age (Busse 1969) and may in turn impair physical health (Lowenthal et al. 1967; Raskind et al. 1974).

An example of age acting as a confounding variable is illustrated in a study of Norwegian concentration-camp survivors who were not studied until about twenty years after their release. These survivors were reported to appear about ten years older than their age. Presumably, undernourishment, heavy labor, and the appalling conditions of the camp, as well as the intense stress of perpetual anxiety and fear, were important etiologic factors. The symptomatology in most survivors included: failing memory and difficulty in concentration, nervousness, irritability, restlessness, sleep disturbances, and fatigue.

Among the institutionalized aged, poor health appears to be significant in predicting whether the individual will successfully cope with major stresses, such as relocation. There is, however, controversy whether this experience does lead to morbidity and mortality. Some have found that relocation has a negative outcome, while others have found no such evidence, or a mixed effect. The poorest candidates for relocation are reportedly those with psychosis, brain impairment, poor mental status, and poor physical functioning (Lawton and Nahemow 1973). Aldrich and Mendkoff (1963) observed that patients became apprehensive when the news of a move was announced; that those who took the move in stride or were overtly angry had the highest survival rate; and that the highest mortality rate occurred among those who regressed, became depressed, or denied that the institution was closing.

Although the data on stress and life crises are still largely descriptive, the results consistently suggest that most healthy aged individuals successfully cope with "on time" stressful situations (Meyer 1974). Although low morale or depression follow traumata, individuals eventually adapt. The effects of repeated encounters with stress over time are less well understood however.

STRESS AND COGNITIVE BEHAVIOR

The relationship between the pathophysiological and cognitive consequences of stress is complex. To date, the findings have been primarily correlational in nature. In 1974 Wang and Busse reported that intellectual impairment as measured by the Weschler Adult Intelligence Scale was associated with both compensated and decompensated heart disease, more so than expected on the basis of the EEG and other reported neurological findings of CNS deficit.

Earlier, however, Busse and Birren, as well as other investigators, reported that no consistent relationship was found between the EEG and psychological test results. This combination of findings would seem to support Birren's discontinuity hypothesis. That hypothesis suggests that variations in cognition remain largely autonomous of somatic functioning until limiting levels are reached, probably as a function of disease. This would predict that there is no simple relationship between advanced age per se and loss until some critical level is reached after which there is a cognitive loss.

In the earlier studies of EEG and intelligence, there was no correlation among normals, but if a normal and a pathological population were mixed, good correlations were achieved. The pathological population (as manifested in both EEG and intelligence) yielded higher correlations, but this was secondary to the discontinuity achieved by adding subjects with CNS pathology, rather than a simple continuum of aging.

Szafran reported in 1968 that the cardiopulmonary status of healthy pilots was related to performance on choice reaction times, sequential decision-making, and a variety of other functions in overload conditions. Spieth's work on pilots (1964) indicated that, with this highly selected population (the average intelligence of pilots is approximately 2 standard deviations above the norm), unmedicated hypertensive pilots did not perform as well as did healthier pilots on intelligence tests. On the other hand, hypertensives whose blood pressure was kept within normal limits by medication performed about the same as normotensives. Spieth also suggested that slowing in reaction time was more likely to occur with decision-making on the more complex problems.

Wilkie and Eisdorfer examined the relationship between blood pressure and intelligence in individuals aged 60–79 residing within a community. They discovered that diastolic pressures of 105 mm Hg or above were related to significant intellectual decline over a ten-year period among those first seen at age 60–69. Those with normal blood pressure showed relatively little intellectual change, and those with mild hypertension improved slightly over a ten-year period. This suggests that Obrist's earlier contention (1964) that mild elevation of blood pressure may be valuable to maintain adequate cerebral circulation among the aged may be a valid hypothesis.

In the Wilkie and Eisdorfer study, among those aged 70–79, none of the hypertensives survived ten years. Abrahams and Birren (1975) discovered that men aged 25–59 who appeared to be free of cardiovascular disease but who were classified as type A, according to the Rosenman-Friedman typology, had longer response latencies. Since type A has been related to neuroendocrine changes, it has been suggested that this profile may relate to cognition. These data thus indicate that diseases of a stress character, and those involving the sympathetic nervous system, *do* lead to some kind of compromise in performance.

We can only speculate on the basis of the findings. Cerebral circulatory insufficiency is the logical prime factor accounting for the association between cardiovascular disease and poorer performance in humans. Since hypertension is often associated with atherosclerosis and heart disease, cerebrovascular insufficiency could well play a significant role in so-called normal cognitive decline of the aged, if indeed normative decline exists. However, for the early stages of essential hypertension and in the absence of atherosclerotic lesions, the suggestion that circulatory insufficiency is the basis for cognitive dysfunction is really less tenable.

According to Forsyth (1974), in the early stages of essential hypertension, blood pressure may be only transiently elevated. On the other hand, there may be an exaggerated fluctuation of blood pressure in response to emotional or environmental stress, since excessive sympathetic nervous system activity is one of the mechanisms in essential hypertension. This would support Speith's contention that the stress of testing might have more impact upon circulatory hemodynamics in hypertensives than in normotensives. That is, there may be a preexistent sympathetic nervous system imbalance in a person who is about to manifest clinical hypertension.

The emerging literature indicates that performance can be affected by stress or heightened arousal level. Although the relationship is a complicated one, it now seems clear that too low an arousal level, as well as high arousal level, produces inefficiency, and that performance may be best at an intermediate level of arousal. Thus, the relationship between autonomic arousal and behavior can be illustrated by an inverted U-shaped curve, with autonomic arousal on the abscissa and performance on the ordinate. This curve is influenced by a variety of variables, including the nature of the stress, the perception of the stress, the nature of the behavior that is present, and the personality of the individual.

Since individuals with cardiovascular diseases often seem more anxious to begin with than healthy individuals, the poor performance observed among persons with cardiovascular disease may in part be due to situational stress exacerbated in the face of pathological changes as the disease progresses.

SUMMARY AND CONCLUSION

There is much data to support the hypothesis that patterns of behavior—including performance on tests of cognitive functioning—relate to ongoing stress, diseases, and pre-disease states, independent of aging. A growing body of evidence is also emerging elucidating the relationship between disease states and situational factors relating to stress. The process by which stress, however initiated, as a transient, psychophysiologic, activating event leads to more permanent destruction in physiological processes, to the point of pathology, is as yet unknown.

Stress as a basis for accelerated aging is also a reasonable hypothesis, but as yet undemonstrated. The implication of a relationship between stress, disease, aging, and behavior clearly is far reaching. It carries with it the potential for intervention not only at the behavioral level but also at the somatic level. Stress is a physiological event with social and psychological antecedents as well as consequences. We are dealing with a riddle wrapped in an enigma wrapped in more of the same. The potential consequences of mediating stress through the life span are fascinating to contemplate.

ACKNOWLEDGMENTS

The author wishes to express particular gratitude to Ms. Frances Lee Wilkie and Dr. Donna Lee Cohen for their assistance in helping to prepare and review this manuscript.

REFERENCES

Aldrich, C. K., and Mendkoff, E.: Relocation of the aged and disabled: A mortality study, J. Am. Geriatr. Soc. 11:185, 1963.

Appley, M. G., and Trumbull R. (eds.): *Psychological Stress* (New York: Appleton-Century-Crofts, 1967).

Atchley, R. C.: Dimensions of widowhood in later life, Gerontologist 15:176, 1975.

Bridges, P. K., Jones, M. T., and Leak, D.: A comparative study of four physiological concomitants of anxiety, Arch. Gen. Psychiatry, 19:141, 1968.

Broadbent, D. E.: *Decision and Stress* (New York: Academic Press, 1971).

Broverman, D. M., Klaiber, E. L., Vogel, W., and Kobayashi, Y.: Short-term versus long-term effects of adrenal hormones on behavior, Psychol. Bull. 81: 672, 1974.

Brown, G. W.: Meaning, Measurement and Stress of Life Events, in Dohrenwend, B. S., and Dohrenwend, B. P.: *Stressful Life Events: Their Nature and Effects* (New York: John Wiley and Sons, 1974).

Busse, E. W.: Theories of Aging, in Busse, E. W., and Pfeiffer, E. (eds.): *Behavior and Adaptation in Late Life* (Boston: Little, Brown and Co., 1969), pp. 11–32.

Caffrey, B.: Behavior patterns and personality characteristics related to prevalence rates of coronary heart disease in American monks, J. Chronic Dis. 22: 93, 1969.

Carp, F. M. (ed.): Retirement (New York: Behavioral Publications, 1972).

Croog, S. H.: The Family as a Source of Stress, in Levine, S., and Scotch, N. A. (eds.): *Social Stress* (Chicago: Aldine, 1970), pp. 19–53.

Dekker, D. J., and Webb, J. T.: Relationships of the social readjustment rating scale to psychiatric patient status, anxiety, and social desirability, J. Psychosom. Res. 18:125, 1974.

Dunbar, F.: *Emotions and Bodily Changes* (New York: Columbia University Press, 1935).

Edwards, M. K.: Life Crisis and Myocardial Infarction. Master's thesis, University of Washington, 1971.

Eisdorfer, C.: Arousal and Performance: Experiments in Verbal Learning and a Tentative Theory, in Talland, G. (ed.): *Human Behavior and Aging: Recent Advances in Research and Theory* (New York: Academic Press, 1968), pp. 189–216.

Eisdorfer, C.: Adaptation to Loss of Work, in Carp, F. M. (ed.): *Retirement* (New York: Behavorial Publications, 1972), pp. 245–65.

Eisdorfer, C., Nowlin, J., and Wilkie, F.: Improvement of learning in the aged by modification of autonomic nervous system activity, Science 170:1327, 1970.

Eisdorfer, C., Nowlin, J. B., and Wilkie, F.: (in ms.)

Eitinger, L.: Acute and Chronic Psychiatric and Psychosomatic Reactions in Concentration Camp Survivors, in Levi, L. (ed.): *Society, Stress and Disease* (London: Oxford University Press, 1971), pp. 219–30.

Ellis, H. C.: *Human Learning and Cognition* (Dubuque, IA: Wm. C. Brown Co., 1975).

Engel, G. L.: *Psychological Development in Health and Disease* (Philadelphia: W. B. Saunders Co., 1962).

Forsyth, R. P.: Mechanisms of Cardiovascular Responses to Environmental Stressors, in Obrist, P., Black, A. H., Brener, J., and Di Cara, L. V. (eds.): *Cardiovascular Psychophysiology* (Chicago: Aldine, 1974), pp. 5–32.

Friedman, M., and Rosenman, R. H.: Comparison of fat intake of American men and women, Circulation 16:339, 1957.

Friedman, M., Rosenman, R. H., and Carroll, V.: Changes in the serum cholesterol and blood-clotting time in men subjected to cyclic variation of occupational stress, Circulation 17:852, 1958.

Froehling, S.: Effects of Propranolol on Behavioral and Physiological Measures in Elderly Males. Ph.D. diss., University of Miami, 1974.

Gerber, I., Rusalem, R., Hannon, N., Battin, D., and Arkin, A.: Anticipatory grief and aged widows and widowers, J. Gerontol. 30:225, 1975.

Groen, J. J.: The Measurement of Emotion and Arousal in the Clinical Physiological Laboratory and in Medical Practice, in Levi, L. (ed.): *Emotions: Their Parameters and Measurement* (New York: Raven, 1975).

Harkins, E. B.: Stress and the Empty Nest Transition: A Study of the Influence of Social and Psychological Factors on Emotional and Physical Health. Ph. D. diss., Duke University, 1974.

Herr, J. J., and Birren, J. E.: Differential Effects of Epinephrine and Propranolol on Shuttle Box Avoidance Learning in Rats of Different Ages. Paper read at the 26th Annual Meeting of the Gerontological Society, Miami, Florida, 1973.

Heyman, D. K., and Gianturco, D. T.: Long-term adaptation by the elderly to bereavement, J. Gerontol. 28:359, 1973.

Holmes, T. H., and Masuda, M.: Life Change and Illness Susceptibility, in Scott, J. P., and Senay, E. C. (eds.): *Separation and Depression*, no. 94 (Washington, D.C.: American Association for the Advancement of Science, 1973), p. 161.

Holmes, T. H., and Rahe, R. H.: The social readjustment rating scale, J. Psychosom. Res. 11:213, 1967.

Holmes, T. S., and Holmes, T. H.: Short-term intrusions into the life-style routine, J. Psychosom. Res. 14:121, 1970.

Janis, I. L.: Vigilance and Decision Making in Personal Crisis, in Coelho, G. V., Hamburg, D. A., and Adams, J. E. (eds.): *Coping and Adaptation* (New York: Basic Books, 1974), pp. 139–75.

Jenkins, C. D.: Psychologic and social precursors of coronary disease, N. Engl. J. Med. 284:244; 307, 1971.

Karki, N. T.: The urinary excretion of noradrenalin and adrenaline in different age groups, its diurnal variation and the effect of muscular work on it, Acta Physiol. Scand. (suppl. 132) 39:7, 1956.

Kenigsberg, D., Zyzanski, S. J., Jenkins, C. D., Wardwell, W. I., and Licciardello, A. T.: The coronary-prone behavior pattern in hospitalized patients with and without coronary heart disease, Psychosom. Med. 36:344, 1974.

Lacey, J. I.: Somatic Response Patterning and Stress: Some Revisions of Activation Theory, in Appley, M. G., and Trumbull, R. (eds.): *Psychological Stress* (New York: Appleton-Century-Crofts, 1967), pp. 14–37.

Lang, P. J.: Fear Reduction and Fear Behavior: Problems in Treating a Construct, in Sklier, J. M. (ed.): *Research in Psychotherapy*, vol. 3 (Washington, D.C., American Psychological Assoc., 1968).

Lawton, M. P., and Nahemow, L.: Ecology and the Aging Process, in Eisdorfer, C., and Lawton, M. P. (eds.): *The Psychology of Adult Development and Aging* (Washington, D. C.: American Psychological Assoc., 1973), pp. 619–74.

Lazarus, R.: Emotions and Adaptations: Conceptual and Empirical Relations, in Arnold, W. J. (ed.): *Nebraska Symposium in Motivation* (Nebraska: University Press, 1968).

Lazarus, R. S., Averill, J. R., and Opton, E. M., Jr.: The Psychology of Coping: Issues of Research and Assessment, in Coelho, G. V., Hamburg, D. A., and Adams, J. E. (eds.): *Coping and Adaptation* (New York: Basic Books, 1974), pp. 249–315.

Lazarus, R. S.: *Psychological Stress and the Coping Process* (New York: McGraw-Hill, 1966).

Levi, L. (ed.): *Society, Stress and Disease* (London: Oxford University Press, 1971).

Levi, L.: Psychosocial Stress and Disease: A Conceptual Model, in Gunderson, E. K. E., and Rahe, R. H. (eds.): *Life Stress and Illness* (Springfield, Ill.: Charles C Thomas, 1974), pp. 8–33.

Levi, L., and Kagan, A.: A Synopsis of Ecology and Psychiatry: Some Theoretical Psychosomatic Considerations, Review of Some Studies and Discussion of Preventive Aspects, in *Psychiatry Part I: Proceedings, Fifth World Congress of Psychiatry* (Amsterdam: Excerpta Medica, 1971), pp. 369–79.

Levine, S., and Scotch, N. A. (eds.): *Social Stress* (Chicago: Aldine, 1970).

Lowenthal, M. F.: Psychosocial variations across the adult life course: Frontiers for research and policy, Gerontologist, 15:6, 1975.

Lowenthal, M. F., and Berkman, P. L.: *Aging and Mental Disorder in San Francisco* (San Francisco: Jossey-Bass, 1967).

Lowenthal, M. G., and Chiriboga, D.: Social Stress and Adaptation: Toward a Life-course Perspective, in Eisdorfer, C., and Lawton, M. P. (eds.): *The Psychology of Adult Development and Aging* (Washington, D. C.: American Psychological Assoc., 1973), pp. 281–310.

Marx, J.: Aging research (II): Pacemakers for aging? Science 186:1196, 1974.

Mason, J. W.: Organization of Psychoendocrine Mechanisms: A Review and Reconsideration of Research, in Greenfield, N. S., and Sternbach, R. A. (eds.): *Handbook of Psychophysiology* (New York: Holt, Rinehart and Winston, 1972), pp. 3–91.

Mason, J. W.: A re-evaluation of the concept of "non-specificity" in stress theory, J. Psychiat. Res. 8:323, 1971.

Mason, J. W.: Emotion as Reflected in Patterns of Endocrine Integration, in Levi, L. (ed.): *Society, Stress and Disease* (London: Oxford University Press, 1971).

Mason, J. W., Wool, M. S., Mougey, E. H., Wherry, F. E., Collins, D. R., and Taylor, E. D.: Psychological versus nutritional factors in the effects of "fasting" on hormonal balance, Psychosom. Med. 30:554, 1968.

Mechanic, D.: *Medical Sociology* (New York: Free Press, 1968).

Mechanic, D.: Some problems in the measurement of stress and social readjustment, J. Hum. Stress 1:43, 1975.

Meyer, G. G.: The Closing of the Cycle: Old Age, in Bowden, C. L., and Burstein, A. G. (eds.): *Psychological Basis of Medical Practice: An Introduction to Human Behavior* (Baltimore: Williams & Wilkins, 1974), pp. 203–14.

Moss, G. E.: *Illness, Immunity and Social Interaction* (New York: Wiley-Interscience, 1973).

Nelson, P. D.: Comment, in Gunderson, E. K. E., and Rahe, R. H. (eds.): *Life Stress and Illness* (Springfield, Ill.: Charles C Thomas, 1974), pp. 79–89.

Neugarten, B. L.: Personality Change in Late Life: A Developmental Perspective, in Eisdorfer, C., and Lawton, M. P. (eds.): *The Psychology of Adult Development and Aging* (Washington, D.C.: American Psychological Assoc., 1973), pp. 311–35.

Neugarten, B.: Adaptation and the life cycle, J. Geriatr. Psychiatry 4:71, 1970.

Obrist, W. D.: Cerebral Ischemia: The Senescent Electroencephalogram, in Simonson, E., and McGavack, T. H. (eds.): *Cerebral Ischemia* (Springfield, Ill.: Charles C Thomas, 1964).

Parkes, C. M., Benjamin, B., and Fitzgerald, R. G.: Broken heart: a statistical study of increased mortality among widowers, Br. Med. J. 1:740, 1969.

Paykel, E. S., Myers, J. K., Kienelt, M. J., Klerman, G. L., Linderthal, T. J., and Pepper, M. P.: Life events and depression, Arch. Gen. Psychiatry 21: 753, 1969.

Rahe, R. H.: Life Change and Subsequent Illness Reports, in Gunderson, E. K. E., and Rahe, R. H. (eds.): *Life Stress and Illness* (Springfield, Ill.: Charles C Thomas, 1974).

Rahe, R. H.: Multi-cultural correlations of life change scaling: America, Japan, Denmark, and Sweden, J. Psychosom. Res. 13:191, 1969.

Rahe, R. H., and Arthur, R. J.: Life changes surrounding illness experience, J. Psychosom. Res. 11:341, 1968.

Rahe, R. H., and Lind, E.: Psychosocial factors and sudden cardiac death: A pilot study, J. Psychosom. Res. 15:19, 1971.

Rahe, R. H., and Paasikivi, J.: Psychosocial factors and myocardial infarction. II. An outpatient study in Sweden, J. Psychosom. Res. 15:33, 1971.

Raskind, M. A., Alvarez, C., Cole, L. A., and Barrett, R. R.: Geriatric Crisis Intervention: The Experience of an Outreach team. Paper read at the Gerontological Society 27th Annual Scientific Meeting, Portland, Oregon, 1974.

Rosenman, R. H.: The Role of Behavior Patterns and Neurogenic Factors in the Pathogenesis of Coronary Heart Disease, in Eliot, R. S. (ed.): *Stress and the Heart* (New York: Futura, 1974), pp. 123–41.

Rosenman, R. H., and Friedman, M.: The central nervous system and coronary heart disease, Hosp. Prac. 6:87, 1971.

Rosenman, R. H., Friedman, M., Straus, R., Wurm, M., Kositchek, R., Han, W., and Werthessen, N. T.: A predictive study of coronary heart disease. The Western collaborative group study, JAMA 189:15, 1964.

Rosenman, R. H., Friedman, M., Straus, R., Wurm, M., Jenkins, C. D., Messinger, H. B., Kositchek, R., Han, W., and Werthessen, N. T.: Coronary heart disease in the Western collaborative group study. A follow-up experience of two years, JAMA 195:86, 1966.

Rosenman, R. H., Friedman, M., Straus, R., Jenkins, C. D., Syzanski, S., Jr., Wurm, M., and Kositchek, R.: Coronary heart disease in the Western collaborative group study. A follow-up experience of 4-1/2 years, J. Chronic Dis. 23:173, 1970.

Sarason, I. G., DeMonchaux, C., and Hunt, T.: Methodological Issues in the Assessment of Life Stress, in Levi, L. (ed.): *Society, Stress and Disease* (London: Oxford University Press, 1971).

Sarason, I. G., and Johnson, J. G.: The Life Experiences Survey: Preliminary Findings, Technical Report SCS-LS-001 (Washington, D.C.: Office of Naval Research, 1976).

Scott, R., and Howard, A.: Models of Stress, in Levine, S., and Scotch, N. A. (eds.): *Social Stress* (Chicago: Aldine, 1970).

Selye, H.: Thymus and adrenals in the response of the organism to injuries and intoxications, Br. J. Exp. Pathol. 17:234, 1936.

Selye, H.: The general adaptation syndrome and the diseases of adaptation, J. Clin. Endocrinol. Metab. 6:117, 1946.

Selye, Hans: *The Physiology and Pathology of Exposure to Stress* (Montreal: Acta, 1950).

Selye, H.: *The Stress of Life* (New York: McGraw-Hill, 1956).

Selye, H.: Stress and aging, J. Am. Geriatr. Soc. 18:660, 1970.

Selye, H.: *Stress in Health and Disease* (Boston: Butterworth, 1976).

Spieth, W.: Cardiovascular health status, age and psychological performance, J. Gerontol. 19:284, 1964.

Stokes, R. G., and Maddox, G. L.: Some social factors on retirement adaptation, J. Gerontol. 22, 329, 1967.

Timaris, P. S.: *Developmental Physiology and Aging.* (New York: Macmillan, 1972).

Tyhurst, J. S.: The Role of Transition States – Including Disasters – in Mental Illness, in *Symposium of Preventive and Social Psychiatry* (Washington, D.C.: Walter Reed Army Institute of Research, 1957), pp. 149–69.

U.S. Public Health Service: Monthly Vital Statistics Report: Summary, 1973, vol. 22, no. 13, 1974.

Vinokur, A., and Selzer, M. L.: Desirable versus undesirable life events: Their relationship to stress and mental distress, J. Pers. Soc. Psychol. 32: 329, 1975.

Wang, H. S., and Busse, E. W.: Heart Disease and Brain Impairment among Aged Persons, in Palmore, E. (ed.): *Normal Aging II* (Durham, N. C.: Duke University Press, 1974), p. 160.

Wittkower, E. D., and Dudek, S. Z.: Psychosomatic Medicine: The Mind-Body-Society Interaction, in Wolman, B. B. (ed.): *Handbook of General Psychology* (New Jersey: Prentice-Hall, 1973).

Woolf, S.: Regulatory Mechanisms and Tissue Pathology, in Levi, L. (ed.): *Society, Stress and Disease* (London: Oxford University Press, 1971).

Wyler, A. R., Masuda, M., and Holmes, T. H.: Magnitude of life events and seriousness of illness, Psychosom. Med. 33:115, 1971.

Discussion I

DISCUSSANT: J. H. ABRAMSON
Head of Epidemiological Studies, Brookdale Institute of Gerontology and Adult
Human Development, and Professor of Social Medicine, The Hebrew University-
Hadassah Medical School, Jerusalem, Israel

AS AN EPIDEMIOLOGIST, my comments necessarily have quite a heavy epidemiologic slant. It is clear that the epidemiologic study of cognitive impairment can have different kinds of uses. On the one hand it provides a measure of the size of the problem and the need for care, and on the other hand it is a method of studying etiology and, in the long run, maybe of finding ways of intervention, especially prevention.

Two types of epidemiologic studies have been mentioned in the chapters presented. One of these is the population-based descriptive study. This is directed toward determining how much cognitive impairment there is in a population, at what ages, and in which subgroups of the population.

While it is helpful to define the patient population and, going beyond patients, to see which people are on the borderline, possibly a more important function of such a study is in relation to the study of etiology. Doctor Terry spoke of the theoretical possibility of a slow virus being involved, and he gave us some very encouraging findings related to the scrapie agent. The study of this kind of virus, epidemiologically or any other way, is notoriously difficult, but at least one of the starting points is to know that there are differences between populations. If one knows that breast cancer has a different distribution in different populations, this gives us some hope for possible prevention. If one knows that the distribution of cognitive impairment is different in different populations, this also gives us hope for prevention, and suggests that environmental factors, among others, may be responsible.

The second type of epidemiologic study is the analytic kind, in

45

which one looks for relationships between cognitive impairment and various other factors. Now, here, there are two main aspects of interest. The first is to learn about factors which are predictive of cognitive impairment. If we can find such risk factors and, possibly going beyond this, if we can find evidence that these factors are modifiable and that by modifying them we can reduce the chance of cognitive impairment, then we have a means of intervention.

Doctor Eisdorfer's discussion of blood pressure and cognitive loss might give such an example; he cited one of his own studies (with Wilkie) in this respect. There is now much evidence that blood pressure control can prevent an appreciable amount of cerebrovascular disease. If it can prevent cognitive impairment as well—and here it doesn't matter whether it is doing so through the mechanism of cerebrovascular disease or not—this is another argument in favor of doing something about hypertension.

One could look not only for predictors of cognitive impairment, but also for cognitive impairment as a predictor of something else. Doctor Kay gave us an example in the data he presented on a memory score as predictive of subsequent death from cerebrovascular disease. If people with low memory scores are a high-risk group, they should be given special care.

I personally believe, along with many others, that everyone with a raised blood pressure, including elderly people, should have treatment. One of the arguments put forward against this is that this is a big job: it is a big load on any health service. For this reason it has been suggested that, instead of treating everyone with a raised blood pressure, treatment should be given to people who are at special risk, and various suggestions have been made about how to select these people. A low memory score on a test such as that described by Doctor Kay may be one way of identifying persons who are at very high risk and therefore in especial need of care.

There are problems in the epidemiologic study of cognitive deficits in the aged. As Doctor Eisdorfer said when he spoke about his follow-up study of hypertension, and as Doctor Kay said when he spoke about his follow-up study of people with a low IQ, one of the problems is that we are studying a process. We're looking at change, and unless you know what kinds of changes there are, the degree of change and the rate of change, you can't really get very far in studying the epidemiology of these conditions. From the practical point of view, this means repeated examinations in the form of a longitudinal study—which is extraordinarily difficult, expensive, and time consuming, and which makes great demands on the population being studied.

Another problem relates to the measurement of cognitive deficit. The types of methodological problems mentioned by Doctor Eisdorfer in relation to the study of stress apply to the study of cognitive impairment also, as we heard from Doctor Kay, who said that only "clinical methods" could give definitive results at this time.

While a skilled professional spending time with the person who is being studied can possibly get definitive results, this strategy has certain disadvantages from the epidemiologic point of view. There is considerable room for variation of response in this kind of personal relationship between testee and tester. Given this individual variation, it becomes extremely important to study the epidemiology of cognitive impairment on a large scale, in big-study populations. It is difficult to find enough skilled people to do this testing, and it is extremely difficult to be sure that they will do it in such a way that their findings can be compared with each other. Over and above the variability of the person's response, there is a great deal of interclinician variation, as every study in the psychiatric field has shown. This, then, is a difficulty in the probably more accurate, but more complicated, "clinical" approach.

The use of simpler techniques presents difficulties of its own. The simplest method is to ask the person about himself—to ask him about his memory; however, we have been told about the problems that this approach involves. One gets relatively soft data. Accuracy may be improved a little by asking questions of a relative, but here a new kind of bias comes in.

The most promising approach—and here Doctor Kay is one of the pioneers—is to develop simple and fairly objective tests. There is much work to be done on these tests. Doctor Kay told us that at present the tests used in Newcastle give good results if account is taken of the patient's background. But a need to take account of education, cultural group, and so on makes it very difficult to use such tests in analytic epidemiologic studies, and in cross-cultural studies especially.

Another problem is to find simple methods which are acceptable to people, which don't make them feel inferior when they are presented with tasks which they think they should be able to do well but find they can't. The measures should be simple but have a high validity and a high reliability. All this is very easy to say, but terribly difficult to achieve. I think it is the burning problem in the epidemiologic study of this condition.

OPEN DISCUSSION

FROM THE FLOOR: My first question is about the use of the name or term "senile dementia." Why do we call the disease "senile dementia"? If we use the term "senile," does this mean that we are thinking that the senile changes of the brain are the cause of the dementia? We don't need to use "senile." We should find another term, but not "senile dementia."

And the second question: What are the relations between chronic mental disease and chronic brain syndrome or senile dementia?

FROM THE FLOOR: At the beginning of your remarks, Professor Terry, you mentioned that you think of senile dementia as a continuing of aging. The course of your lecture showed, I think, very distinctly that we're dealing with two definite pathological entities; idiopathic or Alzheimer-type dementia, and atherosclerotic dementia. Each has a defined pathological picture. How does this square up with the statement that Alzheimer's dementia is a normal change? Or does this answer the question that a resident once asked me: If all geriatric patients live long enough, would they all become demented?

A second question, also to Professor Terry, is: Is there any correlation in other parts of the body to the wasting or neuronal loss that one sees in the brain in patients with Alzheimer-type dementia? For example, can one explain what one sees frequently in clinical practice: the loss of weight and the physical wasting of a patient who is brought in for all sorts of physical investigation? In the last analysis the man is suffering from idiopathic senile dementia, which is probably the cause of the loss of weight. Is there a pathological correlation in other tissues with the loss of neurons seen in the brain?

FROM THE FLOOR: It has been my impression that although patients with Alzheimer's and atherosclerotic dementia may show different clinical pictures during early stages of the disease, they appear to become very similar with time, perhaps three to four years after diagnosis. Could you comment on this?

FROM THE FLOOR: In your population studies, have you found any correlation between chronic brain syndrome and those living in an isolated or a stimulating environment—that is, those living alone or those living with their spouses in a proper family setting?

FROM THE FLOOR: I'm concerned very much with the preoccupation in mental testing as it concerns functional loss and intellectual loss, and also with the relationship between stress and mental-test questioning. I think that when we question a patient in a mental test and look for intellectual loss, we are stressing him, and thereby impairing his performance.

Moreover, what is our purpose in undertaking mental tests if it is not to predict or to encourage productive behavior patterns in old people, behavior based, of course, on what is retained? I would like to ask which mental tests are directed to observing what persons retain of useful mental function, in the presence of a deprived life style, rather than what they lose?

I would also like to mention the work of Bevan in Leeds who has devised a number of useful tasks and one in particular which I find helpful: the birthday-present test. The patient is asked to look at a number of objects and relate these to family members who might be suitable receivers of these as gifts. A camera might be for the teenage son, a powder puff for the secretary, and so on. It introduces a real life situation, motivation, familiar behavior patterns, and is more akin to situations in which older people are actually using adult brains.

DOCTOR TERRY: The first question had to do with the nomenclature. I must say that I regard "senile dementia" as a class term obviously including several sorts of situations, one of which is dementia due to extensive loss of cerebral tissue caused by arteriosclerosis; another type due to a more diffuse change in the parenchyma, which we relate to Alzheimer's disease; a third group possibly due to a variety of toxins; a fourth form due to the occasional neoplasm; and so on. I would agree that we probably ought to specify which one we're dealing with. However, in view of the fact that at least two thirds of patients with senile dementia are cases related to Alzheimer's disease, I would not be surprised if those terms became increasingly synonymous in general use as well as in my own speech.

Now in regard to the pathological entity versus the continuity, I agree that there are perhaps many holes in the hypothesis that this is a continuum rather than a discontinuous process. What I meant was that there is a steadily increasing concentration of changes throughout adult life, these changes being organic on the one hand—visible with the microscope or measurable chemically—and on the other hand apparent to the skilled psychologist. There may well be a continuous correspondence between these changes.

In regard to end-stage similarity, this is true in many diseases where we are unable to differentiate what caused the initiation of the process. This is certainly true of various disorders of skeletal muscle, be they dystrophic or atrophic, neurogenic or myogenic. By the terminal stage they are essentially identical clinically.

In the case of the brain, where we might find infarctions in the brain stem, internal capsules, and the cerebral cortex, the patient will appear quadriplegic, aphasic, mute and unresponsive—similar to the advanced, diffuse, dementing process I have called Alzheimer's disease. It is not the end stage which is definitive; it is the earlier stages.

As to the specific cause of the organic changes, I do not know. As to other organs corresponding to the shrinkage of the brain, there certainly is shrinkage of muscle. It's due to numerous causes: disuse atrophy related to arthritis or bone compression in the vertebral column; malnutrition; neuronal loss in dorsal root ganglia. As to other organs, it has been said that if we were to rely entirely on our livers, we could live something like 750 years. Organ specificity varies widely from species to species.

DOCTOR KAY: I think that, because of the pathological investigations that have shown that there are at least two separate processes going on in the brain, vascular changes and degenerative changes, there has been a move, at any rate in England, to distinguish these conditions as separate conditions: (1) senile or degenerative dementia associated with plaques and Alzheimer-type changes, and (2) the arteriosclerotic dementia or vascular dementia associated with softening. The Alzheimer changes are the pathological basis for most forms of what I call senile dementia.

In attempting to relate chronic brain syndrome to isolation, we found that most of the characteristics of our subjects were the consequences of the brain syndrome rather than the possible cause of it. We did find some sex differences, however. More females with brain syndrome were living on their own, whereas all of the men we identified were living with their families. We assumed that this was due to various factors like the differential rates of removal of people with chronic brain syndrome to hospitals. So we didn't find much evidence that isolation was a factor in bringing about a brain syndrome, although it could make it worse by introducing malnutrition and other problems as complicating factors.

DOCTOR EISDORFER: I believe that with time we will probably employ a new terminology, and I think that, ideally, such terminology should be based on differentiation in etiology. If we understand dementia to refer to a very loose symptomatic description of "cognitive decrement" (a term I prefer), and if we dropped the word "senile," we would probably be much better off. Perhaps one of the most important outgrowths of a meeting like this is that we might individually and collectively come up with a better term. Perhaps we ought never to use "senile dementia" unless it is in conjunction with the terms "Alzheimer's" or "cerebrovascular," or some other modifier.

Regarding the stress of psychological testing, it should be understood that there is good evidence that all examinations, including the physical examination, are a stressful experience for the aged. From the data we get it would appear there is almost nothing we can do without modifying whatever it is we're looking at, to some extent.

In response to the question concerning the relationship between the other categories of chronic mental disease and dementia, there are some data on this, but it depends very much on the kind of mental disease we're talking about. Post and his colleagues from England indicate that depression, if not endemic among the aged, is at least quite frequent, but does not of itself predispose people to diagnosed senile dementia. The suggestion that persons with longstanding schizophrenia and other types of chronic mental illness are particularly susceptible to senile dementia has not been supported. There are problems, of course, of overlapping diagnostic terminology. One issue that confounds the interpretation of behavioral data involves the secondary consequences of long-term institutionalization in relatively understimulating settings.

If we examine the epidemiology of these disorders in terms of living arrangements, I'm sure we all know that the probability of being placed in the custodial care environment is likely to be related to family constellation as well as to disease constellation. Thus, social factors affect behavior and interact with biological factors in influencing the severity of a disorder, as well as its outcome.

One of the great difficulties we encounter in working with the elderly has to do with the self-definition of illness. Busse's study at Duke and the study of Adrian Osfeld in Chicago would indicate that older persons exhibit medical pathology to a far greater extent than they themselves admit to. Often they describe themselves as old, while a physician would describe them as sick. We need always to be concerned about this. Since delivery of health care is in part related to the definition of need, and the definition of need does vary considerably according to the psychological and social situation—or what I choose to call the behavioral ecology—such variables must be understood and taken into account.

Two final comments that I would like to make relate to the importance, but extraordinary difficulty, I think, of doing good epidemiologic work in this field. At this time the investigators in the Framingham study in the United States are spending a considerable amount of time trying to assess cognitive loss. It's very difficult to assess change at a single point in time; since that study has been more than a decade in progress new tests and strategies must be devised for their now aged sample.

I hope we learn more about the cohort effect in this regard. One of the things that may confuse us is that age is no longer a simple variable; it never was, but we now appreciate that analysis and interpretation of data is complicated because, at different phases in the history of man, different kinds of information and different learning strategies were transmitted to people. Those aged who are currently 75 are probably different along a number of dimensions than those now 50 will be in twenty-five years when they are 75, or than people now 25 will be in fifty years when they are 75. Aging is a process—and it must be related to the social and historic setting in which the process occurs.

PART II

4 / Psychological Evaluation of the Cognitively Impaired Elderly

JOYCE PARR SCHAIE, Ph.D.
Postdoctoral Fellow, Department of Psychology, University of California at Los Angeles

K. WARNER SCHAIE, Ph.D.
Director, Gerontology Research Institute, Ethel Percy Andrus Gerontology Center, University of Southern California, Los Angeles, California

THIS CHAPTER is concerned with the extent and limits of the contribution to be made by the clinical psychologist to the diagnosis of cognitive impairment in the elderly, as well as to the careful description of behavioral deficits accompanying such impairment. Such a discussion will need to include a review of some of the general issues one must deal with when one is engaged in the psychological assessment of the elderly. But these general issues need to be examined with special focus upon the problem of cognitive deficit. (For a broader discussion of psychological assessment in the elderly, see Schaie and Schaie 1977.) More specific material will then be presented on a variety of techniques and approaches which psychologists have found useful or which may have promise in work with the cognitively impaired elderly.

SOME GENERAL ISSUES

Clinical psychologists entered the professional scene historically by applying scientific procedures to the formal assessment of behavioral constructs, and established themselves by offering detailed psychometric and other formal assessment procedures. Nevertheless, disen-

NOTE: Preparation of this chapter was facilitated in part by a research fellowship grant #AG 5037–02 and research grant #AG 480–03 from the National Institute on Aging.

chantment with psychological diagnostics occurred in the 1950s when it was discovered that many of the favored techniques lacked validity or appeared to be irrelevant to the kind of questions other mental health professionals wanted psychologists to consider.

In retrospect, it now appears that many of the techniques developed by clinical psychologists may be much sounder than originally assumed. We did not give these procedures a chance to be successful, perhaps because we developed some rather elegant techniques before we knew what kinds of questions ought to be asked.

Practitioners of clinical assessment in psychology today have become considerably more sophisticated. They are now prepared to consider the definition of problems and to predict the likelihood of success of intervention techniques, as well as to apply formal techniques to the evaluation of success in intervention. In particular, we have recognized that the clinical assessment process in psychology must utilize the model of the hypothetico-deductive experiment with an N of 1, namely, the client. This means that in modern clinical assessment we do not give a test battery and then try to figure out what the results mean. Rather, the assessment goals are first defined and expressed in the form of hypotheses about the client's behavior. Appropriate methods including tests and interview procedures are then selected to test such hypotheses. If during this process new "hunches" are discovered, the interpretation must then conform to the limitations of all post hoc analyses. Such "hunches" are then operationalized by alternate assessment procedures, and they too are then formally tested before the clinician proceeds to draw formal conclusions (Sarbin, Taft, and Bailey 1960).

Before the clinical psychologist can design diagnostic strategies capable of testing hypotheses regarding cognitive deficit in the individual elderly patient, he must gain some understanding of the normal level of cognitive function in the elderly. Baseline determinations in the elderly are fraught with the difficulties always encountered when we deal with individuals who are functioning close to their marginal limits (Pfeiffer 1973). In addition, we need to be concerned because the behavior sample apparent in our specific assessment situation may not accurately reflect the aged client's capability in a more naturalistic setting (Gaitz 1973).

Whenever performance baselines are obtained, more extensive behavior samples, including procedures which are sometimes called "testing the limits," may be required to reduce unreliability attributable to the greater variability of the older person. Multiple sampling may also be required because older subjects have been found to benefit much more from practice than do the young (Lehman and Kral 1968). In other words, repeated assessment sessions may be required because our first behavior sample may not really be representative of the performance capability of the older individual.

APPLICABILITY OF CONVENTIONAL TECHNIQUES TO THE AGED

One of the most serious problems in the psychological assessment of the elderly is the fact that, with a few exceptions (e.g., Demming and Pressey 1957), most of our tests, questionnaires, and other procedures were devised either in an educationally oriented context involving constructs important to the behavior of children and the young adult, or were scored according to norms developed to detect psychopathology in an essentially young-adult and middle-aged population. For example, the Stanford-Binet, the Wechsler tests, and such personality inventories as the Guilford and Cattell personality scales were all based on what we know about the behavior of children and young adults. Pathology-oriented techniques, such as the Rorschach, the MMPI, or the Bender Gestalt, likewise, were originally designed with patient populations of young adults in mind. Only as an afterthought, as it were, have norms for older groups been collected for some of these procedures. Further, even though a number of special procedures for aged subjects have been developed in recent years for research purposes, more often than not, no thought has been given to their extension or to provision of norms suitable for clinical purposes.

Before it is possible to apply most clinical procedures to the aged with confidence, it is necessary to consider some general issues of reliability as they affect the transposition of procedures to a client population which differs in level of development from that for which the techniques were originally developed (Oberleder 1967). Next, one must consider the impediments to such application raised by differences in test-taking motivation between young adults and the elderly (Botwinick 1969). Attention needs also to be given to the effect of the high incidence of sensory and motor problems in the aged which may affect the validity of many assessment procedures.

It is often taken for granted by gerontologically unsophisticated clinicians that normative data for young or middle-aged adults can be applied meaningfully to aging subjects, even though such norms would frequently misclassify normally functioning older people as being brain-damaged (e.g., Goul and Brown 1970) or neurotic (Swenson 1961). Some gerontologists, on the other hand, assume that virtually no young adult norms may be applied to the aged, and that the validity of all techniques not developed for the aged is automatically suspect (Oberleder 1964).

Both positions, we think, are naive, but for different reasons. The first position makes a strong assumption that the construct, concurrent, and predictive validity of a measurement instrument remains constant in a wide age range, or, for that matter, in the same age group across individuals with markedly diverse characteristics. The second position is equally mistaken because it assumes that all behavior traits change as a function of age (which is not necessarily true), and that the validity of standard techniques must therefore be impaired.

The question of test validity for the application of psychological assessment techniques to the elderly needs to be considered separately for construct and predictive validity. In the case of construct validity, we must conclude that for the area of intellectual functioning—so important in the assessment of cognitive deficit—it is simply not safe to assume that a given test measures the same construct in the old as in the young. A less obvious aspect of the issue of construct validity of tests for the elderly is that tests age as well as do individuals. Thus, tests which have been constructed for a given cohort in adulthood may conceivably remain valid for that particular cohort, or generation, throughout adulthood, but may not be valid for successive cohorts over the age range for which the test was developed (Schaie 1970, 1974).

To expand upon this point, the reader is reminded that language patterns and problem-solving styles are often formed early in life and are remarkably resistant to change. Indeed, the so-called generation gap is often described as being occasioned because different semantic frameworks are used by successive generations to conceptualize very similar behaviors. As a consequence, it is quite likely that the original version of the Wechsler-Bellevue scale, developed upon samples of young adults in the 1930s, might have greater construct validity for today's aged—the same population upon which that test's norms were developed—than would the more recent revision of the test known as the WAIS. And, as successive test revisions occur, and the phenotypic measures of the constructs to be assessed are changed, each new revision should be expected to yield successively diminished validity when applied to the behavior of the older person.

The goal for most psychological assessment has traditionally been the determination of optimal function in young adulthood. Particular techniques may therefore retain high concurrent and construct validity for the purpose of determining whether or not an elderly client maintains adequate levels of function when compared with *younger* individuals. But construct validity may be quite low when the objective is to assess change of function within the individual.

In contrast to the considerations just mentioned, the predictive validity of psychological assessment instruments is tied directly to the availability of appropriate age-corrected norms as well as to the availability of knowledge about the levels of performance required of an older person in a particular job or life situation. That is, to utilize the client's behavior sample to predict whether the client is on a decrement trajectory ("going downhill") or developing age-related psychopathology we must have accurate information how such a client compares with other normally functioning persons of his generation at a similar age.

Since all age-corrected norms found in the scientific literature have been developed from cross-sectional studies, they are, at least in our opinion, strictly cohort specific, and we are in bad shape so far as knowing whether age norms presented in manuals which are ten or twenty years old have any relevance to the behavior of individuals of that same age at the present point in time. Another problem found with normative tables, when comparison with young adult norms is involved, occurs because older clients routinely have had less education, are at a lower socioeconomic status, and are in poorer physical health than the population upon which the norms have been developed. One cannot really fault the test constructor because it is very difficult to develop normative data which take into account the multiple classifications required to adjust for all these factors. But the clinician will need to be sensitive to these issues and avoid the expectation that an aged client of low socioeconomic status and low level of education, even in the absence of pathology, should function at the level which would be average for a better educated member of a more recent population cohort.

MOTIVATIONAL FACTORS IN THE ASSESSMENT OF THE ELDERLY

The under-use of mental health facilities by the elderly, which has been well documented recently (Lawton and Gottesman 1974), may be related to fears that the services provided will indeed lead to loss of independence and other negative status changes. Participation by the elderly in mental health oriented studies and the incidence of self-referrals may therefore be subject to much more serious selection problems than what would be true among young populations (Atchley 1969).

Most clinical assessments of young adults, moreover, are based upon an interaction between the client and the clinician, both of whom are highly motivated to elicit information which will be helpful to the client. A similar situation might be thought to prevail with the aged self-referred client, but we must take into account the greater cautiousness of the elderly, their not-unrealistic expectation of receiving negative feedback, and the extension of their avoidance behavior in the context of the assessment situation (Furry and Baltes 1973). Nevertheless, such behavior is modifiable when suitable incentives are introduced into the assessment situation (Birkhill and Schaie 1975). Other older clients, by contrast, may over-report symptoms. Complaints may be mentioned which were characteristic of discomfort at some time in the history of the patient's difficulties, even though they are not relevant to the present problem (Denney, Kole, and Matarazzo 1965).

Of even greater concern is the tendency of the young professional observer to attend to his stereotypes about the old rather than to the characteristics of the specific client he is working with (Ahammer and Baltes 1972). Such stereotypes may be reduced if the professional has substantial knowledge of the behaviors to be described. Interestingly enough, information on apparent senile changes reported by family members, for example, seem to be quite accurate and have been found to correlate quite highly with clinical findings (Blessed, Tomlinson, and Roth 1968).

SENSORY AND MOTOR PROBLEMS

In the aged, detrimental findings on intelligence tests, evidence of confusion or reality distortion found by means of projective techniques, random-appearing questionnaire responses, as well as apparent perceptual distortion on visual motor tasks, may all be a function of deficit in peripheral sensory and motor functions rather than being diagnostic of organic or functional pathology. Many clients supposedly having signs of brain damage have been found to be misdiagnosed simply because the client forgot to put on his or her glasses—a matter not always observed by the busy mental health professional.

There are undeniable age changes in the efficiency of visual apparatus which could affect performance on psychological tests. These changes include the decreased transparency of the lens, reduction in pupil size, changes in the vitreous humor, and retinal changes (Corso 1971). Even though the clinical psychologist will not always have available detailed descriptions of the visual changes occurring in his client, he must at least satisfy himself that visual acuity has been corrected to the point where the client can handle test details without significant interference.

Unfortunately many of the traditional questionnaires used in clinical practice are printed in typefaces which will either be impossible for the elderly client to read, or which will introduce distortion, if nothing else, because of simple fatigue. Alternate forms with larger typefaces are thus one of the most urgent needs for many of the commercially published clinical psychological tests.

Similar problems are introduced by the auditory changes which affect even the otherwise well functioning elderly adults (Schaie, Strother, and Baltes 1964), but which are much less likely to be compensated for by suitable hearing devices. The tendency of many older people to attempt to please the professional examiner makes it even more likely that the examiner may be unaware of a client's failure to communicate because he has not heard the examiner's question (Hurwitz and Allison 1965).

And finally, there are more subtle changes in motor coordination and muscular control which will tend to influence test behavior both in terms of the greater response time required, and the tendency to produce motor behaviors which in younger individuals might provide diagnostic clues of pathology, but which in the aged may have much more diffuse origins and therefore lack diagnostic usefulness.

ASSESSMENT QUESTIONS

When a person comes, or is referred, for evaluation the first decision which must be made is to determine what specific questions one should try to answer about that person. Specific tests are limited in terms of the information they can provide, and the clinician's and patient's time and energy must be spent efficiently.

When the questions are related to assessment of cognitive deficit, it may be important to estimate how a person is functioning as compared with a former level. Sometimes the critical question is how one is functioning in relationship to the demands of his or her immediate environmental situation.

There are a number of specific questions which clinical psychologists are prepared to address, though admittedly in varying degrees. The first of these is whether cognitive deficit is generalized or specific; whether many functions are lost; or whether the loss is more selective. A second question is whether the deficit is unstable and therefore is perhaps in process, or has become stabilized. An answer to this question might be useful in suggesting possible causative factors and in suggesting whether or not the loss might be reversible. A third question would be whether attitudinal and/or personality factors are contributing to, or complicating, the deficit. Fourth, it may be asked whether the behavior or behaviors of interest might be amenable to change with training. A related question is whether the person has characteristics which make it likely that he or she could benefit from training. Finally, it may be asked whether counseling or psychotherapy is likely to be helpful.

Information regarding known diseases, accidental trauma, or changes in life situation is helpful in deciding what assessment techniques to use, and what to look for in the test data. For example, if a cardiovascular accident had preceded the testing, one would appropriately focus first on the kinds of deficit present and their relative importance. Second, one might look at attitudes which the patient expresses toward himself as a changed person and at personality factors which would suggest the patient's abilities to cope with the changes. Knowledge of how much time has passed since the accident would help in assessing the stability or reliability of behaviors and in judging the likelihood that reassessment at a later time would provide a useful comparison. On the other hand, if the only known change in the relative recent history was one of life circumstance, such as retirement, living arrangements, or death of a relative or close friend, then one would more appropriately focus first on the assessment of personality or attitudinal factors which might secondarily be producing changes in cognitive functioning.

The specific questions just noted can be addressed with varying degrees of success. The science of prediction for older persons still has a long way to go. Some of what is discussed here refers to what is known and possible. The answers to other questions await the outcome of work already in progress. For some questions, we know what data are needed but the relevant research is yet to be done. Some of the discussion which follows, therefore, is idealistic—but it may well provide some perspectives for future work. In any event, it is important to distinguish among these various levels of knowledge and skill, lest an unrealistic expectation is created of what psychological testing can and cannot provide.

INTELLIGENCE TEST SCORES AND THE ELDERLY

It is important that professional health care personnel avoid the use of such terms as "organicity" or "brain damage." (See Davison 1974; and Matarazzo 1972 for discussions of problems related to such use of these global concepts.) The importance of differentiating among the functional syndromes has been more widely recognized, and while a completely satisfactory classification system has not been achieved, different treatments are prescribed with some success for different disorders. For brain damage, however, the global judgment of organicity or its absence has persisted. The lack of specificity has probably been related to the assumption that not much can be done when neural tissue ceases to function. A finer differentiation, however, could provide hypotheses regarding etiology and regarding the kinds of assets that may still be available. Remaining strengths have all too frequently been ignored when a diagnosis of senile dementia has been determined.

Good validity data are available for test indicators of specific deficit as it relates to lateralization in younger and middle-aged adults (Klove 1974). Tests are used which systematically sample behaviors thought to be controlled by specific brain areas. Unfortunately, however, very little information is available regarding test indications of brain damage in the elderly.

In fact, when the typical elderly pattern of scores on the Wechsler subtests (Botwinick 1977) is compared with scores of chronic or acute, right lateralized, left lateralized, and diffuse brain-damaged adult groups (Fitzhugh, Fitzhugh, and Reitan 1962), the elderly pattern is indistinguishable from the pattern of either the chronic or acute right lateralization patient. If anything, one would expect that advanced age groups would look like a chronic diffuse brain-damaged group. Such is not the case (Schaie and Schaie 1977).

This finding may clarify, however, why instruments such as the modified word learning test (Savage et al. 1973) have been among the more successful discriminators of brain damage in the elderly. Such tests are thought to tap primarily left hemispheric functions. Since the "normal" elderly ordinarily show more right hemispheric deficit (visuospatial performance) than left, a marked decrement in a task involving left hemispheric functions should be clinically significant.

Such a test could identify either generalized or left hemispheric damage. By this logic, false negative misclassification would include persons who have predominantly right hemispheric damage, while the false positives could indicate "functional" interference with verbal ability.

The fact that the usual aging pattern involves a lowering of performance on visuospatial tasks could also explain why serious misclassification of older persons has resulted from use of tests such as the trail-making test (Davies 1968; Goul and Brown 1970), the memory for designs test (Alexander 1970), and the arrow-drawing test (Goodly and Reinhold 1964). Patterns of test data which differentiate general classes of normal elderly from those with brain syndrome have been reported (e.g., Overall and Gorham 1972), but little information is currently available which is more specific.

The block design test is the only one that we have found that can be used to differentiate more specific malfunction in the elderly patient. Measures of competence have successfully differentiated between normal persons and brain injured, but measures of style of performance have also distinguished between right and left hemispheric damage (Ben-Yishay et al. 1971).

There is considerable debate about the usefulness of the Wechsler verbal versus performance discrepancies (Savage et al. 1973; Schaie and Schaie 1977). A number of investigators report a high degree of misclassification of elderly patients with the use of these tests. The comparison we made earlier of Wechsler score changes with normal aging and available brain damage data also suggest serious problems with verbal-performance discrepancy measures. Further, the notion that the vocabulary score can be used as a measure of previous function has limited usefulness; it should be accurate enough to diagnose normal patients and right hemispheric patients, but could not be used if there were a suspicion of left or perhaps even diffuse damage. In other words, if the vocabulary score is high, it can be trusted to indicate good previous function; if it is low, we cannot assume low previous function. At present we must rely on other kinds of information to estimate loss — for example, occupational level and achievement.

More critical, usually, is the question of which functions are still intact and which are deficient. The Wechsler subtests are quite useful for this purpose, and norms for the elderly are available. Savage et al. (1973) concluded from their extensive study of elderly community and patient groups that the use of their test battery, including the WAIS and a number of other measures, could not be justified for diagnostic categorization purposes, but they did find that their tests were quite useful for assessing the *degree* of impairment which accompanied whatever disorder was present. Their monograph provides the most comprehensive test findings for normal and patient elderly groups yet available. Their study, however, did not deal with the question of laterality in the brain-damaged groups they tested.

A number of recent studies with elderly persons use several brief intelligence tests which show high correlation with the WAIS (Ammons and Ammons 1962; Savage et al. 1973). Whether one should use the full WAIS or a more abbreviated, and therefore less fatiguing, measure depends upon the kinds of questions one is trying to answer.

In summary, then, tests that differentiate between normal and pathological functions among young groups cannot be assumed to do so with older persons as well. Validation of existing techniques with older groups is desperately needed. The problem is, first, one of getting sufficient information regarding how normal or well functioning elderly persons score on these tests; and second, of knowing how test scores of older persons correlate with behavior in actual life situations. In any case, general adult norms for chronic diffuse loss simply cannot be used to assess brain damage in the elderly. This is an area in which we know what must be done, but it will take some time to do.

MEMORY, LEARNING, AND PROBLEM-SOLVING

As persons age, memory plays a more significant role in test performance (e.g., Botwinick 1973; Savage and Britton 1968; Savage et al. 1973). A number of investigators have reported memory confounding other measures of cognitive function. Because of this confusion and because memory may be of particular interest in itself, there is a need for independent measures of different types of memory function.

The Wechsler Memory Scale (WMS) has seven subtests which combine to provide a memory quotient or MQ. Factor analyses indicate that WMS taps three kinds of memory function in normal subjects: (1) general retentiveness, (2) simple learning, and (3) associational flexibility (Dujoune and Levy 1971). These authors found further that factorial composition differentiated between normal and psychiatric patient groups. Hulicka (1966) reported that age had a differential effect on the various subtests of the Wechsler Memory Scale, but no age differences were found in the 80–92 year olds studied by Klonoff and Kennedy (1965). While Walton (1958) reported a high percentage of misclassification with one administration of the WMS, he found differences between functional and organic patients after four repetitions of the test. While some problems obviously remain in developing appropriate norms, this test seems worthy of further investigation for usefulness with older groups.

A summary of the literature suggests that, whereas a moderate decrement can be expected with advanced age, a large decrement in performance on the digit span task has clinical significance in the elderly (Arenberg 1973). The clinician must pay particular attention to the mode of presentation, however, as older people do much better when the task is presented auditorily, rather than visually (Taub 1972). Several individual verbal learning tests have been useful with elderly groups. These tests have discriminated between normal and generalized brain-damaged groups (Bolton, Savage, and Roth 1967; Savage et al. 1973), and between persons who are near, and far from, death (Hall et al. 1972; Lieberman and Coplan 1970). Some changes in the cutoff scores for the synonym learning test have been suggested in order to assess brain pathology in the aged (Kendrick 1967). Overall performance on verbal learning tasks has been shown to depend upon whether the instructions were given in a supportive or challenging fashion (Ross 1968).

ATTITUDE AND PERSONALITY MEASURES

Attitudinal and personality measurement techniques have been part of the clinical psychologist's repertoire for many years. Again, however, some changes in traditional procedures will be necessary to provide services to the elderly. Even the Minnesota Multiphasic Personality Inventory (MMPI), a useful and trusted instrument, needs some changes in norms if it is to be used. Studies indicate that responses may be affected by age (Aaronson 1960; Slater and Scarr 1964). The generation or cohort to which the respondent belongs is also likely to affect attitudes held toward deviant behaviors and will therefore influence test responses.

Extensive data on MMPI scores of older persons are available from various sources, and revised norms may become available in the future. It may be, however, that in the long run a new form, or forms, of this test will be considered essential. Investigators differ as to whether the MMPI can be used to assess personality variables in elderly brain-damaged persons (Decker 1969; Pfeiffer 1977). The question raised concerns the reliability of responses. Testing and retesting with the Mini-Mult, a shortened form (Kincannon 1968), would assist in determining the degree of consistency for a particular person.

A number of single scale tests of personality variables have been validated with samples of the elderly. For example, studies of self-administered tests of self-concept (Lewis 1971; Preston and Gudiksen 1966), body image (Conte 1970), and social responsibility (Schaie 1959; Schaie and Parham 1974) are available. The Test of Behavioral Rigidity (TBR) (Schaie and Parham 1975) has norms for persons to age 84, which are age-related and generation-corrected. A number of structured behavior observation schedules are also available which can be used when contact with the person is possible over a period of time, such as during hospitalization (see Salzman et al. 1972 for summary).

Recent literature regarding the use of projective techniques to assess personality in older persons leaves much to be desired, particularly in terms of validity studies, i.e., whether or not the scores describe characteristics which have meaningful correlations in real life. We are not questioning whether or not it is possible to demonstrate such relationships, but are saying simply that such relationships have not yet been demonstrated. Thus far, the only external validity data available for the Rorschach, for example, distinguishes between institutionalized versus noninstitutionalized persons and among socioeconomic status levels (Ames et. al. 1973; Oberleder 1967). Ames' use of the categories of normal, presenile, and senile have met with very mixed reactions (e.g., Oberleder, 1967). Further, hearing impairment has been demonstrated as being related to poorer scoring in older persons (Eisdorfer 1960).

Tests such as the Thematic Appreciation Test (TAT) have been used extensively for research purposes with the elderly to study role image differences with age (see Chown 1968 for review). Validity studies are mixed, but among the aged, TAT did discriminate between persons near, and far from, death (Lieberman and Coplan 1970). Several new tests designed for use with elderly persons are available, but validity data have not yet been presented (Bellak and Bellak 1973; Wolk and Wolk 1971). The limited information available has indicated that aspects of drawings made by older persons simply do not mean the same thing as they do for younger people (Wolk 1972).

BENEFIT THROUGH TRAINING

Assessment questions regarding an individual's ability to benefit from specialized training procedures in an attempt to improve cognitive function are important ones. Some types of learning and performance behavior have been improved in older people through specialized practice and conditioning techniques (Crovitz 1966; Hoyer, Labouvie, and Baltes 1973; Meichenbaum 1972). Gottesman, Quarterman, and Cohn (1973) have reviewed the use of behavior modification procedures with the elderly, and several assessment techniques have been investigated for their potential in predicting change in individuals in such programs (Cautela and Kastenbaum 1967).

Various personality and physiological awareness scales are being investigated for predicting the younger person's ability to benefit from biofeedback training (Bergman and Johnson 1971; Blanchard, Young, and McLeod 1972; Ray and Lamb 1974). The research on biofeedback as a technique for enhancing cognitive function, however, is just beginning (Goldman et al. 1975; Woodruff 1975). Further efforts to develop and validate tests which could assist in appropriate linking of persons and training programs seem critical.

BENEFIT FROM VERBAL PSYCHOTHERAPY

We come, then, to the question of whether counseling or psychotherapy is likely to be helpful. If psychotherapy is viewed as helping a person to develop as realistic a picture of himself or herself as that person can handle, and then emphasizing his or her strengths to deal with oneself and the environment, then a number of writers favor such therapy for the elderly patient, even when brain damage has been diagnosed unequivocally (Goldfarb 1962).

The ego strength scale from the MMPI has been useful with younger groups in predicting success in therapy (Barron 1956). Validity data are not available for older persons, however. Scales which measure cognitive flexibility in the elderly (Schaie and Parham 1975) and those which describe elderly persons' techniques of coping with people and events are available (Messer 1967; Tissue 1971) and might be useful in predicting therapeutic outcome. The validity of these scales for such a purpose has not yet been established, however.

Once one has made the decision to try psychotherapy, the critical questions concern whether individual or group therapy should be recommended. Measures of preferred style of interpersonal interaction might here be useful. There are tests which have been used to assess, in older persons, attitudes which reflect types and degrees of their interaction with other persons (Messer 1967; Tissue 1971). Again, however, studies of validity for purposes of predicting success in psychotherapy are needed.

SUMMARY

In summary, then, some tests have been shown to assist in answering specific questions about the cognitively impaired elderly, but many more still lack norms and validity data. The point of all of this is not simply to sketch a pessimistic picture of the current state of psychological assessment procedures with the elderly. It is, instead, first, an attempt to demonstrate that naive use of tests designed for younger persons may at best be misleading and at worst, very damaging to the elderly clients one is trying to assist. Second, we have raised some cautions and made some suggestions regarding the use of specific tests with older persons. And finally, we have pointed to some further work which needs to be done to provide better clinical services for the elderly.

REFERENCES

Aaronson, B. S.: A dimension of personality change with aging, J. Clin. Psychol. 16:63, 1960.

Ahammer, I. M., and Baltes, P. B.: Objective versus perceived age differences in personality: How do adolescents, adults, and older people view themselves and each other, J. Gerontol. 27:46, 1972.

Alexander, D. A.: The application of the Graham-Kendall Memory for Designs test to elderly normal and psychiatric groups, Br. J. Soc. Clin. Psychol. 9:85, 1970.

Ames, L. B., Metraux, R. W., Rodell, J. L., and Walker, R. N.: *Rorschach Responses in Old Age* (New York: Brunner-Mazel, 1973).

Ammons, R. B., and Ammons, C. H.: The quick test: Provisional manual, Psychol. Rep. 11:111, 1962.

Arenberg, D.: Cognition and Aging: Verbal Learning, Memory, Problem Solving and Aging, in Eisdorfer, C., and Lawton, M. P. (eds.): *The Psychology of Adult Development and Aging* (Washington, D.C.: American Psychological Assoc., 1973).

Atchley, R. C.: Respondents vs. refusers in an interview study of retired women: An analysis of selected characteristics, J. Gerontol. 24:27, 1969.

Barron, F.: An Ego-Strength Scale Which Predicts Response to Psychotherapy, in Welsh, G. S., and Dahlstrom, W. G. (eds.): *Basic Readings on the MMPI in Psychology and Medicine* (Minneapolis: University of Minnesota Press, 1956).

Bellak, L., and Bellak, S. S.: *Senior Apperception Technique* (Larchmont, N.Y.: C. P. S., 1973).

Ben-Yishay, Y., Diller, L., Mandleberg, I., Gordon, W., and Gerstman, L. J.: Similarities and differences in block design performance between older normal and brain-injured persons: a task analysis, J. Abnorm. Psychol. 78: 17, 1971.

Bergman, J. S., and Johnson, H. J.: The effects of instructional set and autonomic perception on cardiac control, Psychophysiology 8:180, 1971.

Birkhill, W. R., and Schaie, K. W.: The effect of differential reinforcement of cautiousness in the intellectual performance of the elderly, J. Gerontol. 30: 578, 1975.

Blanchard, E. B., Young, L. B., and McLeod, P.: Awareness of heart activity and self-control of heart rate, Psychophysiology 9:63, 1972.

Blessed, G., Tomlinson, B. E., and Roth, M.: The association between quantitative measures of dementia and of senile change in the cerebral grey matter of elderly subjects, Br. J. Psychiatry 114:797, 1968.

Bolton, N., Savage, R. D., and Roth, M.: The modified word-learning test and the aged psychiatric patient, Br. J. Psychiatry 113:1139, 1967.

Botwinick, J.: Disinclination to venture response versus cautiousness in responding: Age differences, J. Genet. Psychol. 115:55, 1969.

Botwinick, J.: Aging and Behavior (New York: Springer, 1973).

Botwinick, J.: Intellectual Abilities, in Birren, J. E., and Schaie, K. W. (eds.): Handbook of the Psychology of Aging (New York: Van Nostrand Reinhold, 1977).

Cautela, J. R., and Kastenbaum, R.: Assessment Procedures for Behavior Modification with the Aged, in Proceedings of the 20th Annual Meeting of the Gerontological Society, 1967.

Chown, S. M.: Personality and Aging, in Schaie, K. W. (ed.): Theory and Methods of Research on Aging (Morgantown, W. Va.: West Virginia University Library, 1968).

Conte, H. R.: Studies of Body Image: Body Worries and Body Discomforts, in Proceedings of the Annual Convention—American Psychological Association, 1970.

Corso, J. F.: Sensory processes and age effects in normal adults, J. Gerontol. 26:90, 1971.

Crovitz, E.: Reversing a learning deficit in the aged, J. Gerontol. 21:236, 1966.

Davies, A. D. M.: The influence of age on trail-making test performance, J. Clin. Psychol. 24:96, 1968.

Davison, L. A.: Introduction, in Reitan, R. M., and Davison, L. A. (eds.): Clinical Neuropsychology: Current Status and Applications (Washington, D.C.: Winston, 1974).

Demming, J. A., and Pressey, S. L.: Tests indigenous to the adult and older years, J. Consult. Psychol. 4:144, 1957.

Denney, D., Kole, D. M., and Matarazzo, R. G.: The number of symptoms reported by patients, J. Gerontol. 20:50, 1965.

Dujoune, B. E., and Levy, B. I.: The psychometric structure of the Wechsler Memory Scale, J. Clin. Psychol. 27:351, 1971.

Eisdorfer, C.: Developmental level and sensory impairment in the aged, J. Projective Techniques 24:129, 1960.

Fitzhugh, K. B., Fitzhugh, L. C., and Reitan, R. M.: Wechsler-Bellevue comparisons in groups with "chronic" and "current" lateralized and diffuse brain lesions, J. Consult. Psychol. 26:306, 1962.

Furry, C. A., and Baltes, P. B.: The effect of age differences in ability on extraneous variables on the assessment of intelligence in children, adults, and the elderly, J. Gerontol. 28:73, 1973.

Gaitz, C. M.: Mental Disorder: Diagnosis and Treatment, in Busse, E. (ed.): *Theory and Therapeutics of Aging* (New York: Medcom Press, 1973).

Goldfarb, A. I.: The Psychotherapy of Elderly Patients, in Blumenthal, H. (ed.): *Aging Around the World: Medical and Clinical Aspects of Aging* (New York: Columbia University Press, 1962).

Goldman, H., Kleinman, K. M., Snow, M. Y., Bidus, D. R., and Korol, B.: Relationship between essential hypertension and cognitive functioning: Effects of biofeedback, Psychophysiology 12:569, 1975.

Goodly, W., and Reinhold, M.: The Sense of Direction and the Arrow Form, in Halpern, L. (ed.): *Problems of Dynamic Neurology* (Jerusalem: Hebrew University-Hadassah Medical School, 1964).

Gottesman, L. E., Quarterman, C. E., and Cohn, G. M.: Psychosocial Treatment of the Aged, in Eisdorfer, C., and Lawton, M. P. (eds.): *The Psychology of Adult Development and Aging* (Washington, D.C.: American Psychological Assoc., 1973).

Goul, W. R., and Brown, M.: Effects of age and intelligence on trail-making test performance and validity, Percept. Mot. Skills 30:319, 1970.

Hall, E. H., Savage, R. D., Bolton, N., Pidwell, D. M., and Blessed, G.: Intellect, mental illness and survival in the aged: A longitudinal investigation, J. Gerontol. 27:237, 1972.

Hoyer, W. J., Labouvie, G. V., and Baltes, P. B.: Modification of response speed and intellectual performance in the elderly, Hum. Dev. 16:233, 1973.

Hulicka, I. M.: Age differences in Wechsler Memory scores, J. Genet. Psychol. 109:135, 1966.

Hurwitz, L. J., and Allison, R. S.: Factors Influencing Performance in Psychological Testing of the Aged, in Welford, A. T., and Birren, J. E. (eds.): *Behavior, Aging and the Nervous System* (Springfield, Ill.: Charles C Thomas, 1965).

Kendrick, D. C.: A cross-validation of the use of the SLT and DCT in screening for diffuse brain pathology in elderly subjects, Br. J. Med. Psychol. 40: 173, 1967.

Kincannon, J. G.: Prediction of the standard MMPI scale scores from 71 items: The Mini-Mult, J. Consult. Psychol. 32:319, 1968.

Klonoff, H., and Kennedy, M.: Memory and perceptual functioning in octogenarians and nonagenarians in the community, J. Gerontol. 20:328, 1965.

Klove, H.: Validation Studies in Adult Clinical Neuropsychology, in Reitan, R. M., and Davison, L. A. (eds.): *Clinical Neuropsychology: Current Status and Applications* (Washington, D.C.: Winston, 1974).

Lawton, M. P., and Gottesman, L. E.: Psychological services to the elderly, Am. Psychol. 29:689, 1974.

Lehman, H. E., and Kral, V. A.: Psychological tests: Practice effect in geriatric patients, Geriatrics 2:160, 1968.

Lewis, C. N.: Reminiscing and self-concept in old age, J. Gerontol. 26:240, 1971.

Lieberman, M. A., and Coplan, A. S.: Distance from death as a variable in the study of aging, Dev. Psychol. 2:71, 1970.

Matarazzo, J. D.: *Wechsler's Measurement and Appraisal of Adult Intelligence* (Baltimore: Williams & Wilkins, 1972).

Meichenbaum, D. H.: Training the Aged in the Verbal Control of Behavior, in

Proceedings of the Ninth International Congress of Gerontology, Kiev, 1972.

Messer, M.: The possibility of an age-concentrated environment becoming a normative system, Gerontologist 7:247, 1967.

Oberleder, M.: Aging: Its Importance for Clinical Psychology, in Abt, L. E., and Riess, B. F. (eds.): *Progress in Clinical Psychology* (New York: Grune & Stratton, 1964).

Oberleder, M.: Adapting current psychological techniques for use in testing the aged, Gerontologist 7:188, 1967.

Overall, J. E., and Gorham, D. R.: Organicity versus old age in objective and projective test performance, J. Consult. Clin. Psychol. 39:98, 1972.

Pfeiffer, E. A.: Multiple System Interaction and High Bodily Concern as Problems in the Management of Aging Patients, in Eisdorfer, C., and Fann, W. E. (eds.): *Psychopharmacology and Aging* (Durham, N. C.: Duke University Press, 1973).

Pfeiffer, E. A.: Psychopathology and Social Pathology, in Birren, J. E., and Schaie, K. W. (eds.): *Handbook of the Psychology of Aging* (New York: Van Nostrand Reinhold, 1977).

Preston, C. E., and Gudiksen, K. S.: A measure of self-perception among older people, J. Gerontol. 21:63, 1966.

Ray, W. J., and Lamb, S.: Locus of control and the voluntary control of heart rate, Psychosom. Med. 36:180, 1974.

Ross, E.: Effects of challenging and supportive instructions on verbal learning in older persons, J. Educ. Psychol. 59:261, 1968.

Salzman, C., Shader, R. T., Kochansky, G. E., and Cronin, D. M.: Rating scales for psychotropic drug research with geriatric patients: I. Behavioral ratings, J. Am. Geriatr. Soc. 20:209, 1972.

Sarbin, T. R., Taft, R., and Bailey, D. E.: *Clinical Inference and Cognitive Theory* (New York: Holt, 1960).

Savage, R. D., and Britton, P. G.: The factorial structure of the WAIS in an aged sample, J. Gerontol. 23:183, 1968.

Savage, R. D., Britton, P. G., Bolton, N., and Hall, E. H.: *Intellectual Functioning in the Aged* (New York: Harper and Row, 1973).

Schaie, K. W.: The effect of age on a scale of social responsibility, J. Soc. Psychol. 50:221, 1959.

Schaie, K. W.: A Reinterpretation of Age-related Changes in Cognitive Structure and Functioning, in Goulet, L. R., and Baltes, P. B. (eds.): *Life-span Developmental Psychology: Research and Theory* (New York: Academic Press, 1970).

Schaie, K. W.: Translations in gerontology—From lab to life; Intellectual functioning, Am. Psychol. 29:802, 1974.

Schaie, K. W., and Parham, I. A.: Social responsibility in adulthood: ontogenetic and sociocultural change, J. Pers. Soc. Psychol. 30:483, 1974.

Schaie, K. W., and Parham, I. A., *Manual for the Test of Behavioral Rigidity,* (2d ed.; Palo Alto, Calif.: Consulting Psychologists Press, 1975).

Schaie, K. W., and Schaie, J. P.: Clinical Assessment and Aging, in Birren, J. E., and Schaie, K. W. (eds.): *Handbook of the Psychology of Aging* (New York: Van Nostrand Reinhold, 1977).

Schaie, K. W., and Strother, C. R.: Cognitive and Personality Variables in College Graduates of Advanced Age, in Talland, G. A. (ed.): *Human Aging and Behavior* (New York: Academic Press, 1968).

Schaie, K. W., Strother, C. R., and Baltes, P. B.: A study of auditory sensitivity in advanced age, J. Gerontol. 19:453, 1964.

Slater, P. E., and Scarr, H. A.: Personality in old age, Genet. Psychol. Monogr. 70:229, 1964.

Swenson, W. M.: Structured personality testing in the aged: A MMPI study of the gerontic population, J. Clin. Psychol. 17:302, 1961.

Taub, H. A.: A comparison of young adult and old age groups on various digit span tasks, Dev. Psychol. 6:60, 1972.

Tissue, T.: Disengagement potential: replication and use as an exploratory variable, J. Gerontol. 26:76, 1971.

Uecker, A. E.: Comparability of two methods of administering the MMPI to brain damaged geriatric patients, J. Clin. Psychol. 25:196, 1969.

Walton, D.: The diagnostic and predictive accuracy of the Wechsler Memory Scale in psychiatric patients over 65, J. Ment. Sci. 104:111, 1958.

Wolk, R. L.: Refined Projective Techniques with the Aged, in Kent, D. P., Kastenbaum, R., and Sherwood, S. (eds.): *Research Planning and Action for the Elderly: The Power and Potential of Social Science* (New York: Behavioral Publications, 1972).

Wolk, R. L., and Wolk, R. B.: *The Gerontological Apperception Test* (New York: Behavioral Publications, 1971).

Woodruff, D. S.: Relationships among EEG alpha frequency, reaction time and age: a biofeedback study, Psychophysiology 12:673, 1975.

5 / Senile Dementia and "Pseudosenility": Clinical Diagnosis

LESLIE S. LIBOW, M.D.

Chief, Geriatric Medicine, Jewish Institute for Geriatric Care and Long Island Jewish-Hillside Medical Center, New Hyde Park, New York; and Associate Professor of Medicine, Health Sciences Center, State University of New York at Stony Brook, New York

SENILE DEMENTIA is a major public health problem. Approximately 5% to 15% of all people over 65 years of age residing in the community suffer from this problem (Post 1973). The age group over 80 years has an even higher incidence (Post 1973). Somewhere between one quarter (250,000) and one half (500,000) of the patients in nursing homes have significant manifestations of senile dementia (Redick, Kramer, and Taube 1973). Unfortunately, too little time is spent in properly diagnosing and classifying the mental changes of the elderly. This frequently leads to incorrect categorization of certain changes as "senility" (also called "dementia" or "chronic (organic) brain syndrome"). This diagnosis leads to serious implications. Usually, the individual experiences his loss of rights and liberties and is treated as "incompetent." Permanent institutionalization is a likely result.

The primary care physician's approach to patients whose mental changes suggest cognitive deficit (i.e., memory loss for recent events, disorientation to time, place, and/or self, arithmetic difficulties) requires a thorough medical, neurological, and psychosocial evaluation. This chapter focuses on certain essential aspects of the investigation and classification of these mental changes. These aspects are: (1) appropriate laboratory tests; (2) a new, easily administered mental status evaluation; and (3) differentiation of the "pseudosenilities" from true senility.

75

LABORATORY TESTS FOR THE INVESTIGATION
OF SENILE DEMENTIA

The appropriate tests for the investigation of senile dementia are listed in Table 5–1. They are divided into: (1) basic tests which are necessary in a thorough diagnostic investigation, and (2) elective tests which should be obtained where the clinical situation indicates the need.

The applications of these tests are made obvious in the discussion entitled "pseudosenility" that follows. The goal of the clinical investigation is to highlight the reversible and treatable senile dementias and thus prevent patients who have been described previously as having pseudosenility syndrome (Libow 1973) from being improperly treated and improperly deprived of their therapeutic and basic human rights.

The first four tests listed as electives (skull x-ray, spinal tap, brain scan, and EEG) are done in most investigations of new cases of apparent cognitive loss. The computerized axial transverse tomography (CAT scan) (Baker, Campbell, Houser, Reese, Sheedy, and Holman

TABLE 5–1.–LABORATORY TESTS FOR THE INVESTIGATION
OF CHRONIC ORGANIC BRAIN SYNDROME

1. Basic tests
    a. Complete blood count
    b. Erythrocyte sedimentation rate
    c. Serum Na^+, K^+, Cl^-, BUN, Sugar (SMA-6)
    d. Serum Ca^{2+}, PO_4, liver function tests (SMA-12)
    e. Serum B_{12} and folate
    f. Serologic test for syphilis (VDRL, etc.)
    g. Thyroid function test (i.e., total serum T_4 concentration, T_3 resin uptake, serum-free T_4 and T_3, or PBI)
    h. Chest x-ray
    i. Electrocardiogram
2. Elective tests: Where specifically indicated
    a. Skull x-ray
    b. Spinal tap with examination of CSF (in the absence of papilledema or other evidence of increased intracranial pressure, such as erosion of the dorsum sellae, etc.)
    c. Brain scan
    d. Electroencephalogram (EEG)
    e. Computerized axial transverse tomography (CAT; EMI scanner, etc.)
    f. Isotope cisternography
    g. Cerebral angiography*

*The pneumoencephalogram is intentionally omitted because of its morbidity, especially in the elderly, and because the CAT scan has essentially excluded its need.

1974; Fox, Topel, and Huckman 1975) should also be done, where the test is available. Isotope cisternography is an important test in the diagnosis of normal pressure hydrocephalus (Benson, LeMay, Patten, and Rubens 1970) as is the CAT scan (Baker et al. 1974; Fox et al. 1975). There are occasional cases of apparent senile dementia which warrant the invasive technique of cerebral angiography. Since the advent of the CAT scan, there are practically no situations calling for pneumoencephalography, particularly because of the severe morbidity in the elderly accompanying this technique.

FROMAJE: A NEW MENTAL STATUS EVALUATION TECHNIQUE*

Documentation of mental status function by the primary physician is important for proper diagnosis, classification, and measurement of change. The mental status test described here (Table 5–2) can be performed rather quickly by any clinician and is also a useful self-teaching device. It is common to find some parameters of mentation well maintained, while others have badly deteriorated. Even more impressive is the occasional patient with no errors at all in mental status testing, but who displays an inability to function in the community.

There are many approaches to evaluating mental status, including Perlin and Butler's mental status evaluation (1971), Kahn and Goldfarb's MSQ (1960), and Pfeiffer's short, portable, mental status questionnaire (1975). All three of these approaches focus on memory and orientation, the key factors in diagnosing senile dementia. However, other factors such as reasoning, judgment, emotional state, and overall social functions should also be measured in evaluating mental disorders of the elderly. We have developed an approach covering all these areas of mentation that is easily remembered and rapidly administered and scored. This technique utilizes a mnemonic device, FROMAJE, with each letter representing one aspect of mental function, as listed in Table 5–2. The details of the questions to be asked and the scores to be given for various answers are listed in the same table.

*This portion of the paper is written in collaboration with Allen M. Friedman, a third-year medical student at New York University School of Medicine. Mr. Friedman was the first "inexperienced" interviewer to utilize the quantitative FROMAJE approach in the study of this new instrument as a useful screening technique by nonclinicians. Using FROMAJE to test 21 elderly subjects (13 organic mental syndrome, 9 "normals"), he achieved a concordance of 77% with the clinical ratings of an experienced psychiatrist. In the course of a clinical practice, the FROMAJE used by an "experienced" interviewer in a larger group of patients yields an apparent concordance in the range of 90%.

TABLE 5-2. – FROMAJE TEST*

F = FUNCTION

Refers to an individual's mental ability to adequately maintain himself or herself in community and home. In the case of a patient in a nursing home, the question is whether there is the mental ability to return home and maintain himself or herself. This includes matters of food, shelter, clothing, hygiene, and socially unacceptable behavior (includes wandering in the street, nonpayment of rent, starvation, etc.). This rating refers only to mental strength and competence. An individual with adequate mental capabilities, but physically incapable of maintaining himself or herself at home (e.g., after a stroke, etc.) would be rated as +1 for function.

To properly arrive at this rating, the interviewer must ask the relative, friend, and/or nurse about the patient's mental function in recent weeks or months and combine this information with the interviewer's own impression.

Rating: +1 = Mental function is adequate enough so that no at-home support is necessary.

      +2 = Because of mental impairment, patient will need some at-home support at least part of the day or week (from family, friends, visiting nurse service).

      +3 = Because of mental impairment, patient needs 24-hour per day, 7-day per week, at-home support and supervision.

R = REASONING

Ask person to explain the meaning of a proverb. If unsure whether or not the request is understood or the proverb is familiar, ask another one. If educational or cultural background (i.e., non-English speaking) makes interviewer believe that the person does not comprehend the question, use another proverb or saying that is appropriate to this patient's education and culture (via an interpreter). Assign a rating based on use of an appropriate proverb and language. Sample proverbs: (a) the early bird catches the worm or (b) a stitch in time saves nine.

Rating: +1 = Well explained, with general connotations given.

      +2 = Some semblance of meaning given, but some incompleteness or inability to generalize noted.

      +3 = Completely unable to ascribe any meaning, or giving a totally incorrect explanation.

O = ORIENTATION

If no answer is spontaneously given, then present patient with choices. Thus: Day of week? Is it Monday, Tuesday? Is it June, July, etc.?)

1. Time—Inquire (a) Day of week
             (b) Month and date
             (c) Year

2. Place—Where are you now? (If necessary, present choices: Is this your apartment; your house or hotel; a nursing home or a hospital?)

3. Self—(a) Name
         (b) Approximate year of birth or age

*An easily remembered, rapid mental status test of older patients, emphasizing adequacy of overall function and potential need for increased community support services (or institutionalization). Complete interview format, including instructions for inexperienced interviewer, is available upon request from the author.

(table continued)

TABLE 5-2.—(cont.)

Rating: +1 = Generally accurate with only minor errors in time, place, and self.
   +2 = Significant error in one area: time, place, or self.
   +3 = Significant errors in two or three areas: time, place, and self.

M = MEMORY
   Sample questions:
1. Distant—(a) President of the U.S. during World War II who was in wheelchair? (Ans: F. D. Roosevelt)
   (b) U.S. president assassinated within the past 15 years? (Ans: J. F. Kennedy)
   (c) Where were you born?
2. Recent—(a) What did you have for breakfast today?
   (b) Where were you yesterday?
   (c) Remember the number "8."
3. Immediate—(a) What did I ask you about the presidents of the U.S.?
   (b) What number did I tell you to remember? (8)
Rating: +1 = Generally accurate, with only minor errors in distant, recent, and immediate memory.
   +2 = Significant error in one area: distant, recent, or immediate memory.
   +3 = Significant error in two or three areas: distant, recent, and immediate memory.

A = ARITHMETIC
1. Count from 1 to 10.
2. Count backward from 10 to 1.
3. Subtract 7 from 100.
Rating: +1 = Generally accurate with only minor errors.
   +2 = One significant error.
   +3 = Two or more significant errors.

J = JUDGMENT
1. At night, if you need some help, how do you obtain it?
2. If having trouble with your neighbor, what do you do to improve situation?
3. If you see smoke in a wastepaper basket, what action(s) do you take?
Rating: +1 = Generally sensible response.
   +2 = Demonstrates some poor judgment.
   +3 = Extremely poor judgment.

E = EMOTIONAL STATE
   Observe patient's manner during interview. Ask patient about crying, sadness, depression, optimism, and future plans. Consider the patient's behavior in relation to his or her situation; i.e., some sadness or depression is quite appropriate for a significant illness or loss.
Rating: +1 = Emotional state seems reasonable and appropriate for patient's situation.
   +2 = Extensive or inappropriate depression, or grandiosity, or anxiety.
   +3 = Extremely unreal or inappropriate ideas (delusional or hallucinatory behavior: extreme depression and/or suicidal ideas).

TOTAL FROMAJE SCORE AND INTERPRETATION
1. By the inexperienced interviewer
Score: 7 or 8 = No significant abnormal behavior or mentation
   9 or 10 = Minimal organic mental syndrome (dementia) or emotional illness

(table continued)

TABLE 5-2.—(cont.)

---

11 or 12 = Moderate organic mental syndrome (dementia) or emotional illness
13 or more = Severe organic mental syndrome (dementia) or emotional illness
Thus, in the following example

$$
\begin{aligned}
F &= 2 \\
R &= 1 \\
O &= 2 \\
M &= 2 \\
A &= 1 \\
J &= 1 \\
E &= \underline{1} \\
  & 10
\end{aligned}
$$

the patient would be "rated" as having minimal organic mental syndrome (i.e., score of 10).

2. By the experienced clinician: A subjective overall rating of normal or minimal to severe organic mental syndrome is reached. The FROMAJE responses are recorded for later re-evaluation as to response to therapy and/or time.

3. Patients having difficulties with speech, either expression or words, have dysphasia or aphasia. They cannot be evaluated by the FROMAJE scale.

4. An E (emotional) rating of 3 will produce a total score of +9, even if the patient scores normal (+1) on all of the remaining FROMAJE ratings. Thus, the total of +9, or greater, may be a false positive for senile dementia, but does allow this mental status evaluation to highlight emotional illness.

$$
\begin{aligned}
F &= +1 \\
R &= +1 \\
O &= +1 \\
M &= +1 \\
A &= +1 \\
J &= +1 \\
E &= \underline{+3} \\
  & +9
\end{aligned}
$$

The evaluation of FROMAJE, because of the F functional parameter, takes a little longer to administer than previously described tests. FROMAJE takes approximately 20 minutes for the inexperienced interviewer and 10–15 minutes for the experienced clinician. Unlike some prior tests of mental rating status, the final rating is somewhat more a product of the examiner's subjective assessment, since the rating format is more flexible. Rather than ten standard questions scored plus or minus, FROMAJE is a global interview emphasizing many areas of mentation, including overall social function and emotional state. The ease of remembering and administering this test has brought it into use by all of our medical staff and much of our nursing staff, who generally do not apply the numerical ratings, but rather reach clinical conclusions based on the FROMAJE. Controversies about level of mentation are frequent and, in our view, testify to the usefulness of this test. The numerical score is of more meaning for surveys by inexperienced interviewers of large populations than it is for clinical use by physicians.

PSEUDOSENILITY: ACUTE AND POTENTIALLY REVERSIBLE MENTAL CHANGES

Older people with the mental changes of apparent senile dementia are not necessarily suffering from chronic organic brain syndrome. A study at a municipal hospital of patients over 60 years of age who were admitted to the psychiatric screening ward because of abnormal mental function revealed 13% with acute brain syndrome and 33% with combined acute and chronic brain syndrome (Epstein and Simon 1967). Many of these acute syndromes, listed on Table 5–3, are reversible.

TABLE 5–3.—CAUSES OF ACUTE, POSSIBLY REVERSIBLE, MENTAL CHANGES IN THE ELDERLY*

1. Medications
   a. Errors in self-administration.
   b. Chlorpropamide (Diabinese) causes inappropriate ADH secretion leading to water intoxication.
   c. L-Dopa, indomethacin, steroids can induce psychoses.
   d. All drugs with a primary CNS-desired action, e.g., phenothiazines, barbiturates, tricyclic antidepressants, diphenylhydantoin.
2. Metabolic imbalance
   a. Hypercalcemia secondary to
      (1) Carcinoma of lung, breast, and other tissues.
      (2) Primary hyperparathyroidism.
      (3) Multiple myeloma.
      (4) Paget's disease coupled with immobilization.
      (5) Thiazide administration.
   b. Hypocalcemia secondary to
      (1) Malabsorption states.
      (2) Renal failure.
      (3) Hypoparathyroidism: post-thyroidectomy or idiopathic.
   c. Hyperglycemia
      (1) Easily recognized: ketoacidosis.
      (2) Less easily recognized
         (a) Lactic acidosis; look for the "anion gap."
         (b) Nonacidotic hyperosmolarity syndrome; blood sugar above 600 mg/ 100 ml; serum bicarbonate normal; no urinary ketones.

*Adapted with the permission of the American Geriatric Society from Libow, L. S.: "Pseudo-Senility," J. Am. Geriatr. 12:112, 1973.

(table continued)

TABLE 5-3.—(cont.)

---

    d. Hypoglycemia secondary to insulin or sulfonylureas; not with phenformin (DBI) when used alone.

    e. Hypothyroidism: "subacute" onset; low PBI, serum thyroxine (T_4), T_3 resin uptake, and 24-hour I^{131} uptake by thyroid gland; high SGOT, LDH, and CPK; high TSH if primary hypothyroidism.

    f. Hyperthyroidism: may be present in the elderly as depression and/or apathy; termed "apathetic hyperthyroidism"; may also present as dementia.

    g. Hypernatremia: a hyperosmolarity syndrome secondary to
        (1) Inadequate fluid intake in very ill or disoriented patients.
        (2) Cerebral concussion.
        (3) Iatrogenic factors: administration of hypertonic saline by intravenous or intraperitoneal route or tube feeding of high-protein mixtures.
        (4) Excessive sweating without increased water intake.

    h. Hyponatremia: a hypo-osmolarity syndrome secondary to increased antidiuretic hormone secretion; bronchogenic carcinoma; cerebrovascular accident; skull fracture; postoperative period; etc.

    i. Azotemia
        (1) Worsening of a chronic mild nephritis by a urinary-tract infection.
        (2) Medication-induced dehydration or hypokalemic nephropathy.
        (3) "Obstructive" uropathy
            (a) Benign prostatic hypertrophy.
            (b) Neurogenic
                (i)   Diabetes mellitus.
                (ii) Anticholinergics.
                (iii) Antihypertensives: reserpine, ganglionic blockers, hydralazine.
                (iv) Adrenergics: ephedrine, dextroamphetamine.
                (v) Antihistamines.
                (vi) Isoniazid.
        (4) Potent diuretics causing acute bladder overload
            (a) Furosemide (Lasix).
            (b) Ethacrynic acid (Edecrin).
        (5) Urate precipitation in treatment of lymphoma or leukemia
        (6) Calcium precipitation in hypercalcemia syndromes.

3. Depression or acute emotional stress; usually related to "losses."

4. Nutrition: More than 10% of elderly have simultaneous deficiencies of at least three of four important vitamins: thiamine, riboflavin, ascorbic acid, and vitamin A. Deficiencies may play a role in CNS dysfunction and may be due to inadequate intake, or secondary to chronic illness. Pernicious anemia, too, may have CNS manifestations.

5. Tumors
    a. Intracranial:
        (1) Gliomas 50-60% of all CNS tumors, mostly malignant.
        (2) Metastatic, 20-50%; lung, breast, others.
    b. Remote effects of distant cancers: lymphoma, lung.

6. Hepatic conditions
    a. Cirrhosis; onset between ages 40 and 70 years.
    b. Hepatitis; not uncommon in the elderly.

7. Cardiac conditions
    a. Decreased cardiac output secondary to arrhythmia, congestive heart failure, or pulmonary emboli.

(table continued)

TABLE 5-3.—*(cont.)*

---

b. Acute myocardial infarction; 13% of patients have confusion as the major symptom.
8. Vascular conditions
  a. Transient ischemic attacks and cerebrovascular accidents.
  b. Subdural hematoma; 20% of all intracranial masses in the elderly.
9. Any febrile condition
10. Pulmonary conditions: Chronic lung disease (emphysema) with hypoxia and/or hypercapnia; pulmonary emboli.
11. Postsurgical dementia
12. Post-trauma dementia
  a. Accidents.
  b. Assaults.

---

1. Medications.—Errors by the elderly in self-administration of medication are common and often lead to senile dementia (Schwartz, Wang, Zeitz, and Goss 1962; Libow and Mehl 1970). Chlorpropamide (Diabinese) therapy is sometimes associated with a specific syndrome of water intoxication and senile dementia, since it causes increased antidiuretic hormone activity (Weissman, Shenkman, and Gregarman 1971). L-Dopa, indomethacin, and steroids may produce psychotic behavior. Diuretics may lead to dehydration and mental confusion. All drugs with primary action on the central nervous system (e. g., phenothiazines, butyrophenones, and barbiturates) may cause undesirable acute mental changes, including confusion, disorientation, or wandering.

2. Metabolic imbalance.—Hypercalcemia generally produces lethargy and confusion. Many of the major causes of an elevated level of serum calcium are diseases with a peak incidence in, or close to, late life, e.g., metastatic carcinoma of the lung or breast, primary hyperparathyroidism, multiple myeloma, and Paget's disease. All of these situations may be potentiated by immobilization. Thiazide administration, too, may cause hypercalcemia.

Hypocalcemia in the elderly may present as senile dementia. The hypocalcemia may be related to hypoparathyroidism, malabsorption states, or renal failure. These last two causes are usually obvious, but the diagnosis of hypoparathyroidism is easily overlooked in cases of apparent senile dementia. This is an uncommon syndrome and usually is related to prior thyroid surgery. Rarely, one encounters idiopathic hypoparathyroidism in the older patient.

The more easily recognized hyperglycemic state accompanied by confusion is the ketoacidotic state. Less easily recognized and less common is the lactic acidosis syndrome seen in diabetic patients taking phenformin (DBI) and in patients with tissue anoxia. It is characterized by the absence of ketonemia and the presence of acidosis and an "anion gap" between the sum total of major cations (sodium, potassium) and anions (chloride, carbon dioxide, phosphates). The gap is filled by the undetected lactate (Levitan 1969). Less easily recognized, but more common, is the nonketotic hyperosmolarity syndrome, in which hyperglycemia and confusion occur without any ketosis. The mechanism permitting the blood sugar level to rise well above 600 mg/100 ml without ketonemia is not clear. It is probably related to the presence in the serum of low levels of insulin, as compared with no measurable insulin in the cases of ketoacidosis (Johnson, Conn, Dykman, Pek, and Starr 1969). This syndrome and hypoinsulinemia may also be induced by drugs such as diphenylhydantoin.

Hypoglycemia may occur during treatment with insulin or the sulfonylureas (e.g., tolbutamide, chlorpropamide). It does not occur with phenformin when used alone. A likely setting for this syndrome is one of diminished caloric intake related to physical or mental illness, or reduced hepatic or renal function.

Hypothyroidism has been the classic situation used to illustrate the incorrectly applied label of senile dementia.

Hyperthyroidism in the elderly may present as apathy and depression. These patients also usually have a significant degree of cardiovascular disease, weight loss, long-term symptoms, and small multinodular goiters. This condition has been termed "apathetic hyperthyroidism." Hyperthyroidism may also present as dementia, rather than apathy.

Hypernatremia is another form of hyperosmolarity syndrome. The high concentration of serum sodium may result from: (1) inadequate fluid intake in an ill or disorientated patient; (2) cerebral concussion and a resetting of the brain regulatory centers; (3) iatrogenic factors such as the administration of hypertonic saline during peritoneal dialysis or high-protein mixtures during tube feedings; or (4) loss of water in excess of salt (i.e., sweating) without appropriate thirst to compensate for losses.

Hyponatremia is a hypo-osmolarity syndrome and may be due to increased antidiuretic hormone effect secondary to bronchogenic carcinoma, cerebrovascular accident, skull fracture, any surgical procedure, hypothyroidism, tuberculosis, congestive heart failure, cirrhosis, or medications such as the sulfonylureas or clofibrate (Atromid). Azotemia and uremia may be accompanied by mental changes. Urinary infections may augment an underlying chronic, mild pyelonephritis. Diuretics may lead to dehydration or hypokalemic nephropathy. Obstructive uropathy may occur secondary to benign prostatic hypertrophy, neurogenic disorders such as diabetic neuropathy, or to the use of anticholinergics, antihypertensive agents (reserpine, ganglionic blockers, hydralazine), adrenergics, antihistamines, and isoniazid. Potent diuretics, such as ethacrynic acid (Edecrin) and furosemide (Lasix) may cause acute bladder overloading. Urate or calcium salts may precipitate acutely in the kidney (Schreiner 1971).

3. Depression.—Depression is often difficult to distinguish from chronic organic mental syndrome. The differentiation is crucial, since depression is treatable. Recent losses of relatives, friends, pets, or of status and funds should be sought in the history, as should symptoms of insomnia and hypochondriasis. Untoward reactions to medications such as barbiturates or reserpine may also cause depression. Suicide is an ever-present danger, particularly in older men.

4. Nutrition.—Malnutritional states reflecting the simultaneous deficiency of at least three of four important vitamins (thiamine, riboflavin, ascorbic acid, and vitamin A) occur in at least 10% of older people in the United States, and may be accompanied by mental changes (Brin 1968). Vitamin B_{12} deficiency (malabsorption syndromes or pernicious anemia) may also be associated with mental changes.

5. Tumors.—Intracranial tumors present with mental changes in approximately half the cases. The occurrence of symptoms and signs related to cerebral tumors or subdural hematomas is often delayed because of the increased intracranial space available as a result of the cerebral atrophy in the aged. Thus, papilledema occurs in only 11% of brain tumor cases in the elderly. The brain scan often gives positive results in cases of intracerebral tumor (94%) and of subdural hematoma (86%) (Friedman and Odom 1972). The CAT scan is even more accurate (Baker 1974). Metastatic tumors, originating mostly from lung and breast, account for close to half of all brain tumors seen in a general hospital.

Any malignant lesion originating outside the brain, particularly in the lung and lymphatic tissues, may occasionally produce significant CNS changes. The mechanism may be nonmetastatic, e.g., demyelinization.

6. Hepatic conditions. — Cirrhosis of the liver has its most common onset between ages 40 and 70 (Straus 1971). Hepatitis, too, is not uncommon in the elderly.

7. Cardiac conditions. — Diminished cardiac output, secondary to arrhythmia, congestive heart failure, or pulmonary emboli, is often accompanied by decreased cerebral blood flow, which may lead to a confusional state as the major symptom in 13% of these elderly cardiac patients (Pathy 1967).

8. Vascular conditions. — Vascular syndromes (transient ischemic attacks or cerebrovascular accidents) are well known causes of mental changes. However, subdural hematoma is still easily overlooked in the elderly, just as it is easily overlooked in the alcoholic — because there are apparent "other explanations" for the mental changes, i.e., old age and/or alcoholism. Twenty-one per cent of all intracranial masses in the elderly are due to subdural hematomas, and 69% are due to tumors (Friedman and Odom 1972).

9. Febrile conditions. — Any febrile condition or infection can cause transient confusion and senile dementia.

10. Pulmonary conditions. — Chronic lung disease (emphysema) with hypoxia and/or hypercapnia may be present with cerebral symptoms. Pulmonary emboli may also present as senile dementia.

11. Postoperative senile dementia. — Occasional cases of senile dementia develop following major surgery, especially when it is accompanied by general anesthesia. The mechanism is unknown; only some of these patients have a reversal to their premorbid state, sometimes after several weeks to months.

12. Post-traumatic senile dementia. — The frequent accidents and assaults experienced by the elderly are often accompanied by a surprising mental decline even if unaccompanied by direct head trauma. These senile dementias may revert to normal function in as mysterious a manner as that in which they initially occurred.

CHRONIC AND POTENTIALLY REVERSIBLE MENTAL CHANGES

The common chronic mental syndromes include the depressions, dementias, deficiency states, and alcoholic encephalopathies (Table 5-4). The senile dementias are difficult to distinguish clinically and pathologically. Only about 60% of all cases, at autopsy, show a preponderance of either cerebral arteriosclerosis (30%) or of senile

TABLE 5-4.—CAUSES OF "CHRONIC," POSSIBLY REVERSIBLE, MENTAL CHANGES IN THE ELDERLY

1. Depression: must be aggressively diagnosed and differentiated from organic mental syndrome.
2. Dementias: cerebral arteriosclerotic psychoses and senile psychoses; differentiation is questionable.
3. Deficiencies: vitamin B_{12}, other B vitamins, thyroid hormone.
4. Alcoholism, encephalopathy.
5. Low-pressure hydrocephalus: a syndrome of dementia of rapid onset, ataxia, and incontinence. Differentiation from other causes of dementia and/or hydrocephalus is important since it may be treatable. This is not a common cause of dementia.

dementia (30%), while the remainder (40%) show the morphological characteristics of both syndromes (Lanter and Meyer 1968).

Alcoholism is common in the elderly and one third of older patients considered for commitment to state psychiatric hospitals have a background of excessive drinking (Epstein and Simon 1967).

Low-pressure hydrocephalus is an infrequent syndrome presenting as senile dementia of rapid onset, incontinence, and ataxia, and diagnosed by isotopic cisternography. Differentiation from other causes of senile dementia and/or hydrocephalus may be important because of differences in therapy (Benson et al. 1970).

CONCLUSION

One way to ensure "senility" is to misdiagnose a case of reversible cognitive disorder and consequently treat the patient as a case of chronic organic brain syndrome. The medications and the milieu experienced by patients with the diagnosis of chronic organic brain syndrome will certainly combine to fulfill the prophecy. The clinical rule is to seek out and diagnose the pseudosenilities with the expectation that effective therapy will follow.

REFERENCES

Baker, H. L., Campbell, J. K., Houser, D. W., Reese, D. F., Sheedy, P. F., and Holman, C. B.: Computer-assisted tomography of the head, Mayo Clin. Proc. 49:17, 1974.

Benson, D. F., LeMay, M., Patten, D. H., and Rubens, A. B.: Diagnosis of normal pressure hydrocephalus, N. Engl. J. Med. 283:609, 1970.

Brin, M.: Biochemical Methods and Findings in U.S.A. Surveys, in Exton-Smith, A., and Scott, D. (eds.): *Vitamins in the Elderly* (Bristol, England: J. Wright & Sons, 1968), pp. 25–33.

Epstein, L. J., and Simon, A.: Organic brain syndrome in the elderly, Geriatrics 22:145, 1967.

Fox, J. H., Topel, J. L., and Huckman, M. S.: Dementia in the elderly—a search for treatable illness, J. Gerontol. 30:557, 1975.

Friedman, H., and Odom, G. L.: Expanding intracranial lesions in geriatric patients, Geriatrics 27:105, 1972.

Johnson, R. D., Conn, J. W., Dykman, C. J., Pek, S., and Starr, J. I.: Mechanism and management of hyperosmolar coma without ketoacidosis in the diabetic, Diabetes 18:111, 1969.

Kahn, R. L., Goldfarb, A. I., Pollack, M., and Peck, A.: Brief measures for the determination of mental status of the aged, Am. J. Psychiatry 117:326, 1960.

Lanter, H., and Meyer, J. E.: Clinical and Nosological Concepts of Senile Dementia, in Miller, C., and Ciompi, L. (eds.): *Senile Dementia* (Bern and Stuttgart: H. Huber Publishers 1968), p. 18.

Levitan, H.: Acid-based Balance, in Bondy, P. K. (ed.): *Duncan's Disease of Metabolism* (6th ed.; Philadelphia: W. B. Saunders Co., 1969), pp. 1150–70.

Libow, L. S.: Problems Facing the General Physician and Internist in the Management of the Mentally Ill Elderly, in Pfeiffer, E. (ed.): *Successful Treatment of the Elderly Mentally Ill* (Durham, N.C.: Duke University Center for Study of Aging and Human Development, 1976).

Libow, L. S.: "Pseudo-senility": Acute and reversible organic brain syndromes, J. Am. Geriatr. Soc. 21:112, 1973.

Libow, L. S., and Mehl, B.: Self-administration of medications by patients in hospitals or extended care facilities, J. Am. Geriatr. Soc. 18:81, 1970.

Pathy, M. S.: Clinical presentation of myocardial infarction in the elderly, Br. Heart J. 29:190, 1967.

Perlin, S., and Butler, R. M.: Psychiatric Aspects of Adaptation to the Aging Process, in Birren, J. E., Butler, R. M., Greenhouse, S. W., Sokoloff, L., and Yarrow, M. R. (eds.): *Human Aging: A Biological and Behavioral Study*, no. HSM 71–9051 (Washington, D.C.: U.S. Government Printing Office, 1971).

Pfeiffer, E.: A short portable mental status questionnaire for the assessment of organic brain deficit in elderly patients, J. Am. Geriatr. Soc. 23:433, 1975.

Post, F.: Psychiatric Disorders, in Brocklehurst, J. C. (ed.): *Textbook of Geriatric Medicine and Gerontology* (Edinburgh and London: Churchill Livingstone, 1973), p. 195.

Redick, R. W., Kramer, M., and Taube, C. A.: Epidemiology of Mental Illness and Utilization of Psychiatric Facilities Among Older Persons, in Busse, E. W., and Pfeiffer, E. (eds.): *Mental Illness in Later Life* (Washington, D.C.: American Psychiatric Assoc., 1973), p. 203.

Schreiner, G. E.: Obstructive Nephropathy, in Beeson, P., and McDermott, W. (eds.): *Cecil-Loeb Textbook of Medicine* (13th ed.; Philadelphia: W. B. Saunders Co., 1971), pp. 1210–13.

Schwartz, D., Wang, M., Zeitz, L., and Goss, M. E. W.: Medication errors made by elderly, chronically ill patients, Am. J. Public Health 52:2018, 1962.

Straus, B.: Disorders of the Digestive System, in Rossman, I. (ed.): *Clinical Geriatrics* (Philadelphia: J. B. Lippincott Co., 1971), pp. 183–202.

Weissman, P. N., Shenkman, L., and Gregerman, R. I.: Chlorpropramide hyponatremia: Drug-induced inappropriate antidiuretic-hormone activity, N. Engl. J. Med. 284:65, 1971.

6 / The Medical Practitioner and the Elderly Disturbed Patient

LEON EPSTEIN, M.D.
Professor of Psychiatry and Associate Director, Langley Porter Neuropsychiatric
Institute, University of California, San Francisco, California

THE MAJORITY of the aged with psychiatric disorders live in the community, with a smaller number residing in nursing homes, boarding homes, and other residential care facilities. With few exceptions such elderly patients with age-related psychiatric problems are first brought to the attention of, and treated by, physicians other than psychiatrists—by internists, general practitioners, and specialists in family medicine. More often than with the young, their psychiatric disorders may be related to physical illness or the physical decline associated with aging, as well as to age-related psychological and socioeconomic stress. Relatively few of these patients are subsequently referred to psychiatrists, despite the presence in many cases of obvious, and at times severe, psychiatric impairment.

Many of the patients who present themselves to physicians have somatic illnesses of varying degrees of severity or complain of physical symptoms that seem to have little or no organic basis. Their accompanying mental, emotional, or behavioral symptoms of psychiatric disturbance may be obscured by the signs, symptoms, and complaints of physiological disturbance. The successful treatment of a physical illness may result in substantial clearing of concomitant psychiatric symptoms. Even when there is not clear-cut evidence of specific disease, the nonpsychiatric physician may deal quite effectively with the complaints by the very fact of his spending time with the patient and providing sympathetic treatment for aches and pains.

The great majority of elderly patients seen by the nonpsychiatric physician fall into this broad category. The physician feels comfortable and competent to deal with their problems and to work closely with them, even when it becomes clear that the problems are primarily of an age-related psychobiologic nature that may require continuing attention and care.

When the nonpsychiatric physician does consider the referral of an elderly patient to a psychiatrist, it is likely to be the patient whose continuing physiological complaints seem to have no definite organic basis or who does not respond to the physician's efforts over a period of time, and who continues to show intractable emotional or behavioral reactions. The physician is also likely to refer certain patients whose symptoms are very clearly psychiatric, especially the severely depressed patient, the disturbing paranoid patient, the patient who exhibits severe symptoms of delirium, and the patient who is threatening to others or to himself. These are patients who are not only uncomfortable themselves, but also a source of great discomfort to others. The physician will be especially concerned about the depressed patient who appears suicidal, or a potential threat to others because of paranoid thinking; such patients are most likely to be referred for psychiatric evaluation.

Elderly patients with chronic brain syndromes, even when these are of such severity that the patient must be placed in a nursing home, are rarely referred to psychiatrists. They generally remain under the care of the primary physician, who attends to their physical ailments, supervises their general care, and may prescribe psychoactive drugs for insomnia, depression, restlessness, paranoid or confused thinking, or hypochondria, as may seem necessary, in an attempt to maintain the patient's psychological and social functioning in the nursing home or hospital setting. The psychiatrist may be called upon only in the event of some acute change in the patient's behavior, especially if this change may be disturbing or threatening to other patients or staff members.

In general, the elderly person in the community tends to function adequately, despite even severe health disabilities and unfavorable life circumstances, until there is an event with which he cannot cope, e.g., acute illness, accident, environmental stress such as the loss of a spouse, or a forced move to different living quarters (Simon, Lowenthal, and Epstein 1970).

At such a point, decompensation may occur, and the patient or those involved with him in some kind of care-taking capacity most often turn to a physician. The physician quickly learns that he must consider not only the immediate medical problem that may be present but also the complex and interwoven physical, psychological, economic, and social and family factors that influence the overall functioning of the older person. The physician also soon learns that most of these patients either are not using, or are not acquainted with, support services that may be available, such as visiting nurses, social workers, economic supports, home aids, home visiting services, and other services that may be provided by the community.

The treatment possibilities and the prognosis will vary, depending upon such factors as the patient's history, current mental, neurological, and psychological status; social and economic background; and the personal and social resources available. The planning of short-term and long-term care requires a comprehensive evaluation and assessment of all of these factors and a setting of reasonable goals. For the most part, this is done by family physicians, with little involvement of psychiatrists. With certain patients, goals may have to be limited, but almost always something helpful can be done, and often quite a great deal. The essential first step is to recognize that many of the problems may be approachable and are not the inevitable and irreversible result of old age. The goals of treatment for many patients may include decreasing distress and suffering on the part of the patient; improving behavior, and thus decreasing friction between the older person and those around him; increasing capacity for social interaction; and encouraging activities commensurate with the older person's abilities (Goldfarb 1967). These may be accomplished despite the presence of organic brain syndromes of varying degree.

The clinical picture of confusion, disorientation, depression, and memory loss in an older person whom the physician may see in his office, a general hospital or convalescent hospital, or a nursing home, may be a function of a number of conditions, some but certainly not all of which are related to a chronic organic brain disease (Pfeiffer and Busse 1973). A similar clinical picture, for example, may result from depression, which is certainly the most common psychiatric symptom observed in the elderly. It may be the result of a longstanding psychogenic disorder wherein past lifelong experiences and patterns of reaction and behavior have been carried into old age. The neurotic and paranoid reactions observed in the geriatric patient often are exaggerations of such previous personality manifestations with which he has become less able to cope; or the elderly person may be responding to the stress of acute accumulative losses or an unfavorable environmental situation. Here, differential diagnosis is of paramount importance.

The clinical picture of severe confusion may also, as previously noted, be the result of an acute brain syndrome associated with serious physical illness or passing physiological disturbance. Acute brain syndromes are characterized by a relatively sudden onset and are potentially reversible. They may be the result of such acute factors as infection, heart failure, metabolic disturbances, uremia, liver disease, alcoholism, or vitamin deficiencies; and here the clinician must deal with the causative factor.

The significance of the direct relationship between poor physical health and psychiatric impairment cannot be overemphasized. The elderly generally show decreased physical capacity, loss of strength and vigor, and there is an increased likelihood of chronic disabling illness. There is also an increased vulnerability to serious illnesses related to infection, accidents, malnutrition, or alcoholism. Pressing health needs may often include such simple but helpful features as need for dental care, dentures, eyeglasses, or hearing aids. Multiple illnesses are common in this age group, and there are also serious special problems related to alcoholism, drug dependence, and suicide. Alcoholism is a problem more acute in the United States than in some other countries. In a sample of some 526 consecutive patients over age 60 admitted to a psychiatric ward, it was found that 28% had serious problems involving use of alcohol, although this may not have been the specific factor that brought them in for that particular admission (Simon, Epstein, and Reynolds 1968).

Supportive care and treatment of physical illness, when a chronic physical disability is present, is a most important early step in the treatment of any psychiatric symptoms that are present. In many cases, if treatment for physical illness is prompt and appropriate, the psychiatric symptoms will clear so readily as to become virtually unnoticed. On the other hand, the clearing of the physical symptoms and those of the acute brain syndrome may reveal the presence of an underlying chronic brain syndrome which had previously not been recognized. Whatever the presenting problem, the physician must function as a generalist, attending to physical, psychological, social, cultural, and economic problems in a patient whose adaptive systems may already have been operating close to the limits of their capacity, so that additional burdens placed on these systems may have resulted in symptom formation. It is a truism that a multifactorial approach is required.

Contrary to prevailing folklore, it is remarkable how tolerant a family or others in the older person's environment can be, although the older person may express delusions or other bizarre ideation, may be chronically in poor spirits, cranky and complaining, or forgetful, irrational, or eccentric. All these may be accepted as symptomatic of aging. However, should the person become assaultive, threatening, suicidal, or display such potentially harmful behavior as habitually leaving gas jets unlighted, or become incontinent, there will then be an effort to seek care (Lowenthal 1967). The physician may then be consulted regarding placement in a residential care facility of some kind, if initial treatment does not effectively alter the unacceptable behavior. It is interesting to note that the critical events which will bring someone to attention are often not nearly as serious as the illness itself. For example, an elderly man living alone would only enter his house by a ladder extending to a second-floor window, never through the front or the back door. He would occasionally be seen on all fours nibbling at the grass, but nothing was said until he once put his hand on a little girl's leg. At that point the police were called. Thus, what may bring somebody to the physician's attention may not reflect the severity of the illness, but may represent an event which bothers somebody, whether it be a member of the family or someone in the neighborhood.

The approaches to the treatment of mental illness in other age groups is, for the most part, equally applicable to the aged. Many of these patients can benefit from group and individual psychotherapy, pharmacotherapy, the somatic therapies, and supportive approaches. Tranquilizers, antidepressant drugs, and antipsychotic drugs all have been used effectively in the elderly. Although a number of pharmacologic agents have been used to try to alter the course of chronic brain syndromes, these have been quite disappointing. Lithium carbonate for the treatment of manic states and the phenothiazines for the treatment of paranoid conditions are well established in the elderly. Electroconvulsive therapy, although far less used than in the past, may be the treatment of choice for a limited sample of depressed elderly patients who have failed to improve after adequate trial with other approaches.

Special attention must be given to certain dangers that are inherent in the use of drugs to treat older patients, who are far more sensitive than are younger patients to psychoactive drugs, including both tranquilizers and antidepressants. Medication must be given with close attention to initial low, and gradually increased, doses. Furthermore, the incidence of acute brain syndrome associated with toxic drug reactions is fairly high for this age group. In fact, this is one of the frequent causes for psychiatric consultation.

Psychotherapeutic approaches to the emotionally disturbed older patient, whether individual or group psychotherapy, often serve to direct the patient toward increased interpersonal contacts. Many of these patients are insecure and dependent, and the physician often may fill a "parental" role with them. Without being patronizing, he can offer special interest, protection, and help to these patients. He can with great benefit draw the families of older patients more closely into the treatment situation. The physician who is responsible for the care of a patient in a nursing home can encourage the home to make appropriate use of more intensive activity and group programs and of community volunteers.

In summary, the care of the elderly patient—with multiple physical problems and vulnerability to stress, with the concomitant mental, emotional, and behavioral symptoms so familiar to those who deal with this age group—falls mainly to the "family physician" and makes demands upon him. He is the one most frequently consulted by the elderly patient and his family. The presenting complaint may be a specific physical illness, or vague somatic complaints, or clear-cut psychological and behavioral symptoms. It may even be some obviously nonmedical problem for which the distressed patient or his family is seeking help.

For the most part, the physician feels confident about treating these patients and offering appropriate advice and assistance. And he usually is successful, within the limits imposed by the patient's overall condition and the resources available to him, even in those cases where the problems are primarily psychiatric ones.

Only when the psychiatric symptoms are not responsive to this treatment approach or are of such severity as to require specialized care does the primary physician refer these patients to a psychiatrist. This happens less frequently than one might expect, and probably will occur even less frequently as nonpsychiatric physicians become more comfortable in dealing with more severe psychiatric impairment in elderly patients.

Any physician who seeks to give truly comprehensive medical care to his elderly patients will find himself moving beyond a narrow concept of the physician's role and working within a broader framework within which he will be increasingly responsible for the coordination of overall physical, social, and mental well-being of his patients. In this broader framework, he will develop knowledge and appreciation of the variety of resources available to him, including the experience of professionals in social agencies and the findings of the social and behavioral sciences. He will learn to see beyond the traditionally rather narrow focus of the individual physician.

REFERENCES

Goldfarb, A. I.: Geriatric Psychiatry, in Freedman, A., and Kaplan, H. I. (eds.): *Comprehensive Textbook of Psychiatry* (Baltimore: Williams & Wilkins, 1967), pp. 1564–87.

Lowenthal, M. F.: *Lives in Distress, The Paths of the Elderly to the Psychiatric Ward* (New York: Basic Books, 1964).

Pfeiffer, E., and Busse, E. W.: Mental Disorders in Later Life, Affective Disorders: Paranoid, Neurotic, and Situational Reactions, in Busse, E. W., and Pfeiffer, E. (eds.): *Mental Illness in Later Life* (Washington, D.C.: American Psychiatric Assoc., 1973), pp. 109–44.

Simon, A., Epstein, L. J., and Reynolds, L.: Alcoholism in the geriatric mentally ill, Geriatrics 23:125, 1968.

Simon, A., Lowenthal, M. F., and Epstein, L. J. (eds.): *Crisis and Intervention, The Fate of the Elderly Mental Patient* (San Francisco: Jossey-Bass, 1970).

7 / Information and Referral: Components of Comprehensive Care

CHARLES M. GAITZ, M.D.
Head, Special Clinical Services

ROSEMARY McCASLIN, M.S.W.
Director, Senior Information Service

WELTON R. CALVERT, M.S.W.
Program Specialist
Texas Research Institute of Mental Sciences, Houston, Texas

COMPREHENSIVE CARE of elderly persons requires attention to their psychological, social, and physical needs. Although this precept is, by now, universally accepted, delivering complete health care has proved to be no simple matter. Many communities lack some of the required services. Even in cities in which all of the services exist, fragmented health care and poor coordination between care givers often become obstacles to the elderly person who needs help for multiple problems. If an elderly person does not know about a service, or cannot get to it, or cannot pay for it, the service will not be used.

Generally, persons as they age become more dependent and more needful of support from others. Sometimes this support comes from family members, but often the elderly person in an urban industrial community lacks familial support and must rely on social agencies for assistance. Paradoxically, it is in the urban community, where the network of services is so complex, that older people are more likely to give up in frustration. Even younger family members may lack the knowledge and skill to navigate through multiple, sometimes redundant, programs. Persons trained as advocates and coordinators are often needed to provide direction.

DEVELOPMENT OF INFORMATION AND REFERRAL SERVICES

Many communities in the United States have attempted to ease these problems by establishing information and referral services as components in the spectrum of health and social services. The Administration on Aging (AOA) of the United States Department of Health, Education, and Welfare has recognized the importance of such services and has mandated Area Agencies on Aging to establish information and referral services as a first priority in their regional plans. What is an information and referral service? AOA has broadly defined information services as those which:

maintain current information with respect to the opportunities and services available to older persons, and develop current lists of older persons in need of services and opportunities; and employ a specially trained staff, including bilingual individuals as appropriate, to inform older persons of the opportunities and services which are available, and assist them to take advantage of such opportunities and services. (*Federal Register,* October 11, 1973.)

Referral services are defined as those which:

assist individuals to identify the type of assistance needed, place individuals in contact with appropriate services, and follow up to determine whether services were received and met the need identified; and which provide for the maintenance of proper records for use in identifying services offered and gaps in existing services systems. (*Federal Register,* October 11, 1973.)

These services have been operated in various ways: (1) as an office equipped with computer terminals giving access to a complete file of agency data; (2) as an integral part of a social service or health agency; (3) as an attachment to traditional reference sources such as libraries. Whatever the setting, information and referral workers are often viewed as if they were secretaries equipped with a dog-eared copy of the Yellow Pages. There was a time when one called the telephone company and the operator answered, "Information." Now even the telephone company, having renamed the service "Directory Assistance," apparently recognizes that a telephone number is a limited offering and that providing "information" involves much more. Giving a telephone number to a client who wants assistance with locating a nursing home or a doctor is only the beginning.

FUNCTIONS OF INFORMATION AND REFERRAL

Many elderly persons recognize signs of distress; they may also be able to define some of their problems, but they often do not know where to turn for help. As more and more services develop — many categorical, and with differing eligibility requirements — the elderly person may face an overwhelming task in attempting to discover the appropriate agency to meet his or her needs. An information and referral (I & R) service can be extremely useful to such persons, provided that those who staff the service recognize the need for a probing and relatively broad inquiry to determine the caller's needs. A person who contacts an information and referral service stands at the threshold of social service and health care delivery systems. A threshold is a point of departure, a place to begin. An information and referral service provides a central door through which the elderly person can enter many other doors.

The information and referral worker, in addition to directing the client to the agencies best able to serve him or her, can act as an ally — an advocate — in facilitating actual delivery of service. Quite often this involves scaling the tasks involved in applying for assistance to a size that is manageable for a given elderly individual.

Some clients may need encouragement and the support of a worker at an information and referral unit before they are willing to accept a referral. A client's fears may need to be allayed before he or she will go to a health agency or to a psychiatric clinic. There are, of course, persons who need only a minimal amount of service which can be offered directly, without referral elsewhere. For example, we have found that 40% of our I & R clients required referral to only one agency. Directing a client to a welfare agency for financial assistance or to an office to obtain adequate housing may be enough help so that the individual can then deal with other potentially disabling or distressing problems.

It is the responsibility of the information and referral worker, however, to be sensitive and curious; a request for information should not be accepted at face value. Callers often approach the information and referral worker with a request for help with a concrete problem such as transportation, but when given an opportunity, they begin to share many other concerns (Calvert and McCaslin 1972; McCaslin and Calvert 1975). Experience dictates that each client's situation be thoroughly evaluated before a referral is made.

An information and referral service provides a *nonthreatening* point of entry into the service delivery system. This entry point is not labeled "charity" or "mental health" or any other term that may be unacceptable to many of today's elderly. It is labeled, simply, "information" — a door which anyone may open without loss of self-esteem.

PART OF COMPREHENSIVE CARE

An information and referral service may contribute significantly to the client's ability to obtain, and an agency's ability to deliver, some features of comprehensive care. Psychiatrists and social workers long ago agreed that the first interview is critically important in a therapeutic relationship for establishing rapport, clarifying chief complaints, and examining expectations of the patient and attitudes of the care giver (see, for example, Gill, Newman, and Redlich 1954; Roberts and Nee 1970). Yet "intake" functions are often denigrated or ignored. Intake, the initial interview, downgraded as "screening," often is used to protect the clinician or the agency. Too often it is used to determine alternatives so that the client will not have to be seen again.

It is at this very point of contact with an agency that an individual may be most receptive to intervention: the client's discomfort is at its peak, as is the desire to alleviate that discomfort. The individual will begin to move toward a resolution of the problem that will return him or her to a degree of stability. But since the level of adjustment is dependent on whether the person has made a maladaptive or adaptive resolution, intervention should make a major difference.

Perlman (1968) emphasized that persons seeking help are especially sensitive to experiences at the time they acknowledge a need. It follows, then, that an intake worker in a social service agency has a very important function, and that the function is analogous in many respects to that of an information and referral worker. Perlman (1968, p. 171) has described the responsibility of an intake worker as follows:

. . . to bring a person who needs and wants help to the point where he perceives what help is available for his problem, what possibilities, limits, and conditions are involved, what he may expect and what may be expected of him as a participant, and then to come to mutual agreement as to where and how he and the caseworker can move ahead

Perlman's analysis underscores that the worker must be skillful, but does not conclude that a particular professional background is necessary for successful intervention. The effectiveness of intake and referral is dependent on the worker's appreciating the special needs of a person seeking entry into the system and understanding as well the capabilities of professionals to whom a person in need might be referred.

Why should information and referral functions not be given the same recognition and importance as the initial interview with a psychiatrist? And why should this important function not be an integral part of a single agency offering comprehensive care? An effective, integrated information and referral unit removes many of the obstacles of fragmented services. Because the information and referral worker is a member of an agency's team, intra-agency referrals are usually easier than referral to other agencies which may or may not accept a referral. On the other hand, when an interagency referral is necessary, it is facilitated because the information and referral service is backed by the reputation and sanction of the larger agency.

AN OPERATIONAL MODEL

These principles have been applied in developing a model for the delivery of services to elderly persons at the Texas Research Institute of Mental Sciences (TRIMS). Though the program was established in a psychiatric facility, provisions were made for a variety of services by combining an information and referral service and an after-care/alternate-care component with traditional outpatient and inpatient services. These are all components of a single geriatric service headed by a psychiatrist. Psychiatric evaluation and treatment are carried out by a team consisting of a psychiatrist, nurse, and social worker. The information and referral and after-care/alternate-care components are staffed by professional and paraprofessional social workers, including part-time field workers, some of whom are as old as the clients they serve. The service is designed to utilize the special skills of each profession represented on the staff and to facilitate the formation of various treatment teams, based on the needs of individual patients. Each staff member communicates a clear picture of the services he or she can provide, and training at all levels emphasizes the importance of bringing in other team members to augment one's own skills.

The traditional psychiatric components serve elderly persons who have identified emotional problems by providing psychiatric, social, and physical health evaluations and treatment to individuals and families. Both inpatient and outpatient services are available.

About 200 clients are seen on an outpatient basis each month, including about 20 new cases. Inpatient services are provided each year for 55–65 patients, whose average length of hospitalization is about 30 days. During its first year and a half of operation, the evaluation and treatment component reduced geriatric admissions to the state hospital in Harris County from 60 to 20 per year.

The after-care/alternate-care unit deals with elderly persons who

have a history of institutionalization, or who are at risk of institutionalization, to promote participation in a therapeutic program, to assist in
relocating elderly persons in environments that meet their needs, and
to mobilize community resources for secondary support. Many of
these individuals have been referred directly for after-care/alternate-
care. The workers in this component rely on the particular abilities of
staff working in the traditional psychiatric component, and approximately 50% of the patients are referred to the clinic. Conversely, a
significant number of persons seen initially in the clinic or hospital
are referred for services provided by the after-care unit.

The primary recipients of the information and referral service are
elderly persons who have had little or no previous contact with a mental health system. Regular coverage by the media increases community awareness and encourages utilization of this service. The information and referral workers guide clients in coping with personal
problems, assist them in identifying and using resources, and facilitate their entry into the TRIMS' geriatric program. Information and
advice is also given to relatives, professionals, and other concerned
individuals, but whenever possible, staff members talk directly with
the older person involved in an effort to deal with the situation from
the client's point of view. All clients receive at least one follow-up call
a month after the initial contact, but many clients are followed more
closely to provide support in time of crisis and to motivate the individual to accept the services of an appropriate agency.

Three to four hundred persons have contact with the information
and referral service each month, including 50–100 persons having no
previous contact with any part of TRIMS' geriatric service. Over 400
referrals are made monthly for a wide variety of services, the most frequent being for assistance with medical, dental, mental health, and
financial problems. As expected, many people whose first contact with
TRIMS is through the information and referral service do not require
the services offered by the other components.

USE OF THE TELEPHONE

Questions may be raised about the potential problems of providing
services via the telephone. Persons who do not have telephones may
be unable to reach the service. It has been our experience, however,
that most people have access to a phone—their own, or they will use a
neighbor's telephone, or a pay phone to call us. Fieldworkers sta-

tioned at community-based senior centers reach still other persons who need our services.

Another limitation of telephone contacts is the loss of subtleties of communication, such as body language, that are important in interviewing. Experience and training in telephone interviewing techniques can compensate for this disadvantage to some extent. A worker using a telephone learns to ask questions that are unnecessary in face-to-face interviews (e.g., "Are you able to walk without assistance?"), and becomes more attuned to nuances of verbal expression, the meaning of silences, and other differences.

On the positive side, a telephone service is welcomed by individuals who prefer anonymity. The person on the other end of a telephone line may remain a stranger or become a friend, as the caller wishes, and for some persons this situation offers freedom to express needs and feelings that might remain hidden in face-to-face contact. (For further discussion of the therapeutic use of the telephone, see Lester and Brockopp 1973.)

SUMMARY

Mental health care, especially for elderly clients, must have a broad base and approach; a narrow theoretical concept will fail. Mental health professionals more and more acknowledge that obtaining food stamps and providing transportation and adequate housing are important therapeutically. Providing such secondary support is an important function of an information and referral service. For some clients, the provision of these services may prove to be more decisive than evaluating defense mechanisms and modes of coping, and may prevent the development of serious problems.

Information and referral can be an easily identified, nonthreatening service for elderly persons at a time when they are most anxious and most highly motivated to solve their problems, and at the same time least able to sort through a maze of services alone. It can be a service that is sensitive to the client's needs and will supply him or her with appropriate assistance. Information and referral also functions as a preventive mental health service by providing assistance in the resolution of social and environmental problems that may have an adverse bearing on the older person's mental health and, in this process, can bring to light more complicated emotional and psychiatric problems. In the delivery of comprehensive care, information and referral services provide primary care and facilitate coordination with more traditional services.

REFERENCES

Calvert, W. R., and McCaslin, R.: Central intake: Coordination or confusion, Gerontologist 12:73, 1972.

Gill, M., Newman, R., and Redlich, F. C.: *The Initial Interview in Psychiatric Practice* (New York: International Universities Press, 1954).

Lester, D., and Brockopp, G. W.: *Crisis Intervention and Counseling by Telephone* (Springfield, Ill.: Charles C Thomas, 1973).

McCaslin, R., and Calvert, W. R.: Social indicators in black and white: Some ethnic considerations in the design and delivery of services to the elderly, J. Gerontol. 30:60, 1975.

Perlman, H. H.: *Persona: Social Role and Personality* (Chicago: University of Chicago Press, 1968).

Roberts, R. W., and Nee, R. H.: *Theories of Social Casework* (Chicago: University of Chicago Press, 1970).

U.S. National Archives and Records Service: *Federal Register,* vol. 38, no. 196 (Washington, D.C.: U.S. Government Printing Office, October 11, 1973), title 45, chapt. 9, section 903.2.

Discussion II

DISCUSSANT: E. W. BUSSE, M.D., SC.D.
Dean of Medical Education, Duke University Medical Center, Durham, North Carolina

I WOULD LIKE TO BEGIN my comments with the need to merge social and health information and services. I think all of us who work with the elderly realize at some point how closely the social stresses, the economic problems, and the health problems of the aged merge.

At Duke University we have attempted to put together a comprehensive service for the elderly. In doing so we have encountered some very interesting and serious problems. One of them is the matter of record-keeping. For a physician to make good evaluations he needs social data. There is a problem of confidentiality, and we have discovered that some of the information that is given health personnel such as the physician or the nurse may be used differently by other people in the broader network, and the patients involved get very concerned when they discover that other people have this information. We have even discovered that other agencies outside of the University structure wanted some of the data that we had gathered in order to make judgments which, in our opinion, might have been adverse to the health of the individual. How do we, then, develop an adequate record system that is truly useful to all and yet protects the confidentiality of certain items which do seem to be the province of some, particularly the psychiatrist or those in the area of mental health, who can really use them effectively?

Another general question is why those of us who are interested in the elderly are often not well accepted in the teaching framework. And why is it so hard for us to get service programs going? Is there a negative attitude toward the elderly?

We have attempted to identify those patients whom the house staff and students are most likely to dislike. The first group is not the elderly but the very obese; they generate the most negative reaction. The

105

second group is the known long-term hypochondriac; if house staff know them, they really are unhappy to see these patients coming into the clinic. Another problem group is the younger individual who has a chronic disability which is the result of an accident which is probably his own fault, e.g., those who are paraplegics as a result of having been engaged in activities of a questionable nature. Medical students and house officers do not like them. Then you move to the next group: students and residents are uncomfortable with many elderly people; they particularly don't like chronically ill elderly people, and often they get their feelings toward the elderly mixed up with their negative attitude toward the hypochondriac. So then we are faced with the situation that there are elderly people who are disliked by those who take care of them. The next question is: why don't they like them? And: can we possibly change this attitude?

I believe that a major problem lies in the fact that the patient groups I've cited are those least likely to show improvement. The issue, then, is that in order to treat them effectively we have to alter the value system. And we even have to alter the reward system for the caretakers involved, and this really requires some structural changes. It needs to be done very gradually but purposefully.

Doctor Epstein brought up the fact that the physician ought to be aware of the social support systems, and should be capable of referring patients to them. In our experience, the physician who takes a great deal of time referring his patients to the social support systems finds that he gets pressured, and frequently reports that he does not believe that he is distributing his time properly.

So what do you do? You find a very skillful person, a psychiatric nurse or a social worker, and ask him or her to be the liaison person who implements and really makes these contacts. But here again we found a defect; most people are unwilling to do this job for more than two to three years, and then we find that their reward system runs out. They say: "I'm tired of doing this; I want to get back to really helping someone, and being someone in it." We've had this problem with a very skillful social worker. She does this very effectively, but we really have to work on her to keep her in the position; we have to make sure she gets her rewards in some way. So we have to consider the personal needs of the individual who is doing this job, and work to really make him or her content and effective.

To move on to the next issue, I was very intrigued with the problem of evaluation of perceptual skills and cognition. It is of great importance to do evaluations effectively. I do feel that the emphasis which *was* made, and I was very pleased to hear it, was one of looking at perceptual skills. It is amazing to me how often this is overlooked. Often older people are not adequately judged because one is not considering their levels of visual or auditory capacity.

I am particularly struck by the fact that very few examiners seem to realize that it is very important for an older person to have a bright light, and that older persons require an increased intensity of illumination in order to see and perform at the same task as effectively as a younger person; nor do examiners seem to realize what defects in hearing do to functioning, and how often an older person, when he does not understand the full sentence, will actually interpret a word, just a single word, in a different way, producing unbelievably different results.

I also want to refer back to Doctor Kay who described a very brief procedure for evaluation of brain function, utilizing ten questions. To develop comprehensive care it is necessary to have an evaluation system. However, the socioeconomic levels of the patients must be considered when devising brief evaluation systems. Furthermore, simplified procedures should correlate reasonably with the total capacities as judged on the Wechsler Adult Intelligence Scale.

Finally, I have a comment about stress. I've been interested in stress, and particularly interested in the hypochondriacal person. We've known, at least from our longitudinal studies, that if a woman—particularly a woman—is exposed to a social stress of a particular type, i.e., one in which she is very highly criticized, and especially if she is criticized for those roles which have been important to her self-esteem, for example, her role as a mother or as a home carer, she is likely to react and employ hypochondriacal defenses.

Recently I have had the opportunity to review older patients in our newly established family care unit. I have been observing the hypochondriacal older people in this setting. There appear to be more women than men, but I have found that there is a different social problem in this group as compared with the group we studied longitudinally. The difference has been that the most likely social stress that we find among these persons is that of a woman taking care of her husband who may not really deserve being taken care of. He has decided that he isn't going to work very much any more, that he is sick. He may become hypochondriacal and overemphasize his disabilities. She in turn starts falling into the same pattern, and starts utilizing the health care services as a major means of support.

We did find in our longitudinal studies that the resolution of the social factor resulted in the disappearance of the hypochondriacal symptoms. Consequently the person got well with no medical intervention. Clearly, hypochondriasis can come and go, depending upon how intense and acute the social stress may be.

OPEN DISCUSSION

FROM THE FLOOR: I would like to contribute a few points. The first is that the labeling of older persons according to one or another professional bias has almost passed. The second is that evaluation and diagnosis is necessary; and the third is that psychological tests, which for partly justified as well as unjustified scientific reasons became discredited in the United States during the early 1960s, are returning in more sophisticated forms. Finally, I think it is an important point that Wechsler, at the end of his life, wrote that the term "cognitive functioning," so widely used since the Americans discovered Piaget, refers to only part of the total functioning of a person. This is particularly true, I think, for the elderly.

FROM THE FLOOR: I was glad to hear the comment about alcoholism in the aged. In a study I participated in, in Britain, we found that alcoholism was often missed as a diagnosis on admission to hospitals because it was an occult diagnosis and often obscured by physical disease. It is one of the very important points in geriatrics to think of this diagnosis.

FROM THE FLOOR: When one thinks of the people who require custodial care, who in fact should take care of these people? Should they be in a geriatric setting, or in a psychiatric setting, or should they be in a custodial setting? When McCune in 1960 reviewed the disposition of the mentally disabled elderly, he found it was a question of whatever place had a bed available.

DOCTOR EPSTEIN: In response to the question: who should provide custodial care, it might be stated that this issue is in a state of flux. In the state of California, for example, the determination was made to close the large state hospitals for the mentally ill, and offer care in the local community. The state hospitals had ranged in size from about 1500 to about 7500. Although there was merit to the concept, the change was made before many local communities had time to set up programs for the large number of people who would be cared for in the community.

State hospital patients were discharged into a variety of alternative settings. Some went into hotels; others into family care homes, where a caretaker or family might take care of as many as eight persons. Some of these settings were very appropriate and offered excellent care. Others were absolutely inadequate in that patients simply sat in isolation. A number of elderly patients are in nursing homes, many of which, because of insufficient funds, have difficulty providing a program of meaningful comprehensive care.

In summary, there does not appear to be a single best setting within the limits of available funding. Realistically, placement tends to be made where vacancies exist in any of these settings, and where an attempt is made to offer comprehensive care within their funding limitations.

I would also like to comment about labeling, which has great impact not only on the nature of treatment but also on how the person himself responds to that label. This may be a very powerful force for each.

DOCTOR GAITZ: I would like to make a point about responsibility. We started out some years ago with a concern about comprehensive care and a multidisciplinary team as a mode of delivery service; we started out with the notion that every member of the team would do what he could do best. And it became clear very quickly that physicians were not going to do the things that they could, by training and position, do. So we gave up this idea, and proceeded then to assign responsibilities to what we called coordinators: nurses, social workers, and others.

I think this is important because, if we go on with the notion that things ought to be the way they *ought* to be, this extends then to where people should be treated: nursing homes take responsibility, state hospitals take responsibility—*everybody* takes responsibility on paper. When they don't want to do what they are responsible for doing, that's when we get into trouble. So the issue of where should old people be cared for seems to me to be an irrelevant question. The question is: Who is going to take the responsibility and actually do anything?

DOCTOR EPSTEIN: You are indeed correct in your statement that it is not so much a question of which place is most appropriate, but rather, is the particular place, irrespective of its designation, a good place? There are times when a nursing home is an excellent place if it is operated by people who are able to take advantage of all available support systems and who are tremendously interested in their patients. Other nursing homes which do not share these values may not be appropriate. The same applies to hospital settings, family care settings, or indeed the patient's own home.

Thus, it is not the name one gives the setting, or the titles of those in charge, but rather a question of who will take responsibility and how does that person deal with the responsibility assumed?

PART III

8 / Comprehensive Care of the Cognitively Impaired Elderly

BERNARD ISAACS, M.D., F.R.C.P. (GLASGOW), M.R.C.P. (EDIN-BURGH)
Charles Hayward Professor of Geriatric Medicine, University of Birmingham, Birmingham, England

THIS CHAPTER deals with "comprehensive" care, using the expression in its two meanings: giving all the care that is needed, and giving care to all who need it.

In the United Kingdom, with a population of 55 million, about 5% of our people are aged 75 and over, and nearly 1% are aged 85 and over. According to Doctor Kay's figures 10% of those aged 75–84 and 20% of those 85 and over exhibit senile dementia. This means that there may be as many as 350,000 individuals who have senile dementia in our population. We have fewer than 200,000 psychiatric hospital beds, more than half of which are occupied by patients under the age of 65 and about half of the remainder by those aged 65–74. So only about one quarter of our aged with senile dementia are accommodated in psychiatric hospitals. Of the remainder, some are under close supervision in geriatric hospitals and in residential homes (roughly equivalent to American nursing homes), and the others live at home.

Elderly people with senile dementia need to be under constant close supervision; otherwise they may do grave damage to themselves or to others. Much of their care necessarily falls upon those aged 45 to 64—the daughters, the nurses, the home helps, the volunteers, the neighbors who assist them. If we take the ratio of population aged 45 to 64 to that of the population aged 75 and over, we arrive at what one might term a "geriatric care index." Table 8–1 shows the value of this index as it is at present, as it was in the recent past, and as it is expected to be in the future. As recently as 1931 the ratio was 12 middle-aged people to one aged 75 and over. By 1951 the ratio had

TABLE 8-1.–POPULATION RATIO OF
MIDDLE-AGED TO OLD–UNITED KINGDOM

YEARS	AGED 45–64 (MILLIONS)	AGED 75 AND OVER (MILLIONS)	RATIO
1901	5.6	0.5	13 :1
1931	9.8	0.8	11 :1
1951	12.7	1.8	7 :1
1971	13.7	2.6	5 :1
1991 (Projected)	12.8	3.3	3.5:1

fallen to 7:1; in 1971 it was 5:1; and in 1991 it will be 3.5:1. The data also show that for every 6 old people in the United Kingdom in 1971, there will be 8 in 1991; but for every 6 people in the age group 45 to 64 in 1971 there will be only 5 in 1991. The explanation is that people in the United Kingdom now entering old age come from the generation preceding the First World War, when the birth rate was high. But they derive their support from the generation born after the First World War, when the birth rate was low. In all countries with a like experience, such as the United States, a similar increasing disproportion between the old and the middle-aged may be anticipated.

With more people to care for and fewer people to do the caring, we have to devise a new system of care in order to achieve the comprehensiveness that we seek. But who wants to do this kind of work? In the United Kingdom a band of psychiatrists within the Royal College of Psychiatry have formed themselves into a group who are especially concerned with the psychiatry of old age. The formation of this group was strongly encouraged by the first president of the Royal College, Sir Martin Roth, and it is now under the distinguished leadership of Felix Post. The group numbers 120 psychiatrists, some of whom care exclusively for the elderly, while others profess a major interest in the psychiatry of later life. This nuclear group represents only a fraction of the psychiatrists working in mental hospitals who care for the elderly among others, and I have been told by several of them that their interest is in "mainstream" psychiatry. But if half of their beds are occupied by old people, is not mainstream psychiatry minority psychiatry?

Some psychiatrists have also told me that elderly patients with mental failure should not be in psychiatric hospitals; they should be in geriatric units. But already in geriatrics departments, a high proportion of the patients suffer from mental impairment. Geriatric physicians accept this as part of their commitment, and struggle to give the best service they can; but with limited resources and insufficient nursing staff, the geriatrician fears that if he devotes his resources to patients that he cannot cope with, he will have nothing left for those with whom he can cope.

The type of problem we face is illustrated by a patient seen recently. She was a lady of 89 who had been widowed for 15 years and who had shown progressive intellectual change for the previous 7 years. She lived alone. She derived some help from neighbors and from her only son who visited her as often as he could. She was managing to cope despite increasing loss of memory and concentration. Then her dog was killed, and, as her son said, that "snapped the chain." That was the last of a long series of losses and stresses to which she had been exposed. At that stage her behavior became irresponsible, to the point of shocking and horrifying her neighbors. She took off all her clothes and wandered out into the street. This is one of the frontier posts of the land of senile dementia, the point where behavior moves from the tolerable to the unacceptable. The pressure mounted; something had to be done. I was called to see her. She was dressed only in an old dressing gown that was not even properly tied. As I spoke to her she took a paper tissue out of a packet, held it in front of an electric fire that was itself dangerously wired, slowly and inaccurately lit a cigarette, and then threw the lighted tissue onto the carpet. This was another signpost to the territory of senile dementia. The fears of her neighbors overcame their compassion. She had to be "put away" — not because she was ill, but because she was dangerous and unpleasant.

For people such as this we have the alternatives of admission to hospital, where we do not have sufficient beds, or leaving them at home, where we do not have sufficient services. In the United Kingdom it has become fashionable to talk of "community care," as though this was something different from looking after old people at home. A great deal of help, to be sure, is given by our statutory and voluntary domiciliary services; but this help is intermittent, while the hazards of dementia are continuous. "Community care" frequently involves straining the tolerance of relatives and friends beyond endurance.

MODELS OF ILLNESS

Until recent years the minds of doctors and laymen were attuned to an "acute" model of illness. When people became ill, they either died or they recovered. Both the external structure of health care, the "acute" hospital, and the internal structure of human emotions reflected this pattern of illness. When people were ill, their relatives felt compassion and concern. When patients recovered, relatives were gratified; if they died, sorrow and regret were felt. The pattern was right; people were attuned to it emotionally; the social system required and accepted sacrifice; and relatives were glad to give it.

Through improvements in sanitation, immunizations, and antibiotics, as well as other social and medical advances, we have noted marked shifts in the nature of patterns of illness. Acute diseases have become a diminishing portion of health care. Increasingly the medical scene became dominated by long-term, chronic, disabling illness. After a period of adaptation, a health care system was invented to meet chronic illness. This was by no means perfect, but the concept of geriatric medicine was developed, with its emphasis on rehabilitation, social assessment, and multidisciplinary care. The situation of the chronically ill patient was not always irretrievable or hopeless. Within a pattern of multiple disability, there was nearly always something which could be identified and improved. In the United Kingdom this model of management of chronic illness is beginning to gain ground. Doctors and nurses are being attracted into the practice of geriatric medicine. Relatives and social services pitch their expectation of need toward the realization of this concept of long-term care.

A major threat to the health care delivery system of every Western country is the new problem of the vast population of older people with senile dementia. There is no suitable model of illness for them because by and large they are not ill. In this third model, the patients are sad cases or just nuisances. Many of them are awkward, nasty, disgusting, filthy people, a distortion of their original personalities. The geriatrician has few more poignant experiences than when a daughter comes to him and says, "Doctor, that is not my mother." She is expressing in a word the sadness, the guilt, and the emotional turmoil which she experiences because she can no longer relate to the person whom she once loved. We as doctors have just as much difficulty as she has as a daughter in getting our emotions right toward these patients.

Just because I practice geriatric medicine, I do not feel myself bound to like all old people. Some can be cruel; they can hurt and manipulate those who devote themselves to their care. One old lady of 92 who was not even ill, just lonely and insecure, compelled her widowed daughter, a nursing sister aged 55, to sacrifice her professional work and her opportunity of obtaining a pension on retirement in order to come and live with her. The old lady required her daughter to be in bed with her every night at 8:30 P.M. She never allowed her to go out or to live any life of her own. This manipulative old lady poisoned the life of her daughter. Relatives like this daughter live in a state of emotional turmoil, where one half of them wants to discharge their obligation of duty toward their aged parent, and the other half hates this caricature of a once-loved parent, who will leave nothing but unhappy memories of years of barren and futile servitude.

Sons and daughters cannot relate to their cognitively impaired parents; and doctors and nurses have similar difficulties in relating to these patients. Psychiatrists, trained to understand human beings, seem to experience special difficulty in understanding the distortions of human beings caused by senile dementia, and look in vain for opportunities to deploy their special skills. I feel that some psychiatrists have not acquired the sense of commitment that is necessary to perceive that the psychiatry of old age means more than the management problems posed by the patient's immediate symptoms, but that it includes the need to relate this clinical picture to the previous life and personality of the victim; to understand how this deterioration is seen by the relatives; and to come to grips with their own feelings and those of their staff when faced by senile dementia. These psychiatrists are missing the opportunity to interest themselves in psychiatric material of great richness. And how can we hope to develop truly comprehensive care for this group of patients until psychiatrists accept this problem as part of psychiatry?

ORGANIZATION

In the United Kingdom, responsibility for the care of elderly with senile dementia is shared between psychiatrists and geriatricians. When both are under pressure of resource shortage, as is generally the case, there is a danger of each discipline expecting the other to take responsibility for the patient. This is divisive and harmful to patient and profession.

May I draw an analogy from the world of commerce? We have in the United Kingdom a very successful retail chain called Marks and Spencers, which sells clothes and also sells food. This firm did not divide the population into those who want to buy clothes and those who want to buy food and provide one shop for each. They created one shop, with a clothes department and a food department, and a staff who could work in either. They decided not to cater separately for clothes customers and for food customers, but just for people. Some people who came into the shop to buy clothes might buy food; and some who came in for food might also buy clothes.

Now Marks and Spencers is a very successful organization, so the principle was obviously correct. And if it is correct in shops, why is it not correct in hospitals? The present system of separate psychiatric and geriatric services, as Parnell has said, is designed to cater to "mindless bodies" and "bodiless minds." Instead, a service is needed that caters to *people*. This can be achieved by collaboration between psychiatrists and geriatricians, and there are many successful examples of such collaboration in the United Kingdom. However, it is not happening in most areas yet, partly for administrative reasons, and partly because the professions involved still have some difficulty in finding, in their own areas, colleagues who think along similar lines.

SPECIALIST UNITS

Specialist units, admirable though their intended use may be, are not necessarily the best models on which to develop a comprehensive service nationally. Specialist units depend on special motivation, and do not transplant to areas where motivation runs at an average level. Where no joint psychogeriatric assessment services are offered, elderly patients with mental illness may enter the hospital system purely at random through one of many different portals — and may never reach a unit organized to give them the care which they need.

A possible model for future development is that which exists at Hollymoor Hospital, Birmingham, England, where the local geriatric physician has a substantial holding of beds in the mental hospital. These are additional to his main stock of beds, which is in a modern department of geriatric medicine in a general hospital. The geriatric physician is not responsible for all the elderly patients in the mental hospital. Most of these are looked after by psychiatrists. Nor does he remove all elderly patients with mental abnormality from his own main geriatric unit to his beds in the psychiatric ward. This would be divisive and unrealistic; and his staff in the geriatric unit are well accustomed to managing moderately severe mental illness in the elderly. But they are protected from caring for the most demanding patients, such as those who tend to wander, and who seem to do much better under the care of mental hospital nurses. At the same time, he brings a physician's eye to bear on problems in the mental hospital which are not wholly psychiatric. Most important of all, the presence of the geriatric physician in the psychiatric hospital offers an opportunity for day-to-day informal contact, mutual participation, and collaboration in educational and research activities. Ideas, attitudes, and techniques are shared; each branch of the profession becomes more self-sufficient; a wide range of facilities—including outpatient, day-patient, and "outreach" services—is made available to both disciplines, and greater readiness develops to accept a commitment to this group.

This is but one system of care that has been developed to face the third model of illness. It will expand to provide counseling services for relatives; discussion groups and other self-educational activities for nurses and rehabilitation personnel and for social workers; and an active approach to physical diagnosis and rehabilitation. If, in addition, there is in every academic center a University Department of Geriatric Medicine and a University Department of Psychiatry actively collaborating in the education of medical undergraduates and of physicians, psychiatrists, general practitioners, and community physicians, then the real problems of this third model of illness will be identified, studied, and taught. If comparable developments take place in the nursing and social work professions—and in the thinking of social service, housing, and employment departments—then we shall move toward truly comprehensive care of the vast numbers of old people with cognitive loss who will be our future patients.

9 / Nursing Care of the Cognitively Impaired Aged

MIRIAM J. HIRSCHFELD, R.N., M.S.
Tel Aviv University, School of Continuing Medical Education, Department of Nursing;
and Kupat Holim, Dinah School of Nursing, Beilinson Medical Center, Tel Aviv,
Israel

WORKING WITH PEOPLE who have become cognitively impaired is difficult. But it is not impossible, and improvements in their ability to function can be achieved.

A change in mental status is the most common early symptom that something is going wrong with an aged person (Agate 1971). Planning care requires that the care givers be aware of the aged person's ability to cope with stress, that they assess his physical state as well as his psychological and social resources. The impact of age-related losses of health, income, employment, social status, spouse, and peers also must be evaluated. Each of these factors can cause cognitive impairment or add to it.

Myra Levine's (1973) four principles of conservation are useful in deciding what will help the cognitively impaired aged person, and determining what the priorities should be in his or her care:

1. Conservation of energy. The ability of the human body to perform the work of life depends on its energy balance—the supply of energy-producing nutrients measured against the rate of energy-using activities. The nurse acts as a "banker" for the proper balancing of the patient's energy account. She provides for an adequate deposit of energy resource and carefully regulates the energy expenditure.

2. Conservation of structural integrity. This is the necessary de-

Originally published as "The Cognitively Impaired Older Adult." Copyright December 1976, The American Journal of Nursing Company. Reprinted from American Journal of Nursing vol. 76 no. 12.

fense of anatomical and physiological wholeness, the basis for a multitude of nursing interventions.

3. Conservation of personal integrity. For every individual, his sense of identity and self-worth is the most compelling evidence of wholeness. It is the individual life experiences that come out of a person's cultural and historical background that enable him to identify himself as a unique person. Nursing care must conserve and promote this personal integrity.

4. Conservation of social integrity. A human being's social integrity is tied to his family and friends, to the viability of his entire social system. Nursing care must provide optimal social integrity for the individual, with a commitment to health care delivery to his social group as well as to all members of a society when they need such care.

These four principles can be adapted to the care of the cognitively impaired adult so that his remaining capacities are kept intact and used.

CONSERVATION OF ENERGY

An insufficient supply or inefficient utilization of oxygen and glucose cause or contribute to many brain disorders (Wang 1969). A medical diagnosis guides the nurse in assessing how acute a situation is, the likelihood of sudden change, and the prognosis.

The vital signs of a confused patient with suspected increased intracranial pressure, for instance, guide one in finding the optimal balance between rest and activity. Symptoms of anemia, dehydration, electrolyte imbalances, and vitamin deficiencies will determine what diet a patient should be given as well as how much energy he can expend.

Mr. L., 72 years old, was diagnosed as having senile brain disease. Always an active man, Mr. L. knew every tree in his orchard, and for years he walked his 30 acres daily. But when he developed congestive heart failure, his energy level decreased. Still, he would attempt his daily walk, but brain disease had destroyed his sense of orientation. The orchard had become a labyrinth to him, and he could not find his way.

His distressed family would find him among the trees, confused and worn out. Fearful that he might break a leg, they watched him during the day, locked the doors and windows at night. Mr. L. grew more restless, pacing his room at night so that no one got much sleep.

Drugs were tried with no success. Then a nurse suggested that someone walk with him each day in the orchard, letting him lead and taking a folding chair so he could rest. He would have exercise and be doing something that had been meaningful to him all his life. It worked: he seemed happier, and less confused, and he slept at night; the household was no longer on guard.

Anxiety changes energy requirements. Knowing a person's anxiety level and reducing high levels is a prerequisite for increasing available energy.

For example, Ms. G., an 82-year-old, frail lady, was hospitalized with a concussion from a fall. She was desperately lamenting the death of a son 60 years ago. Her anxiety was so overwhelming and her current, actual, and anticipated loss so painful, that she could not face the present.

By listening to her, holding her, bathing and feeding her, encouraging her to rest, we, over time, helped Ms. G. to focus on her present concern: "My husband is 87. How is he managing? He has diabetes and his legs are so bad. I am the one who takes care of him. He is alone at home, I am so scared—perhaps he is dead. I miss him so terribly; I want to see him!"

The nurses persuaded her living son to bring his father for a visit. The day after the visit, she was able to feed herself and walk to the bathroom. A week later, her physical condition so improved that she was nearly independent.

She smiled and then took my hand. "You know, now I am not confused, but I could feel it. There was nothing to hold on to and I just did not know, didn't know. It happens to my husband. Now I can see how he loses his mind and how he is getting nearer to death. Tomorrow I fear it is me."

Helping her work through her past unresolved grief let her resolve her confusion and allowed her to regain energy to cope with the impact of her physical injury (Lindemann 1965).

Kahn (1971) and others describe depression as resembling organic brain disease, for with it comes motor retardation and disturbances in sleep patterns. Conveying to an older person that he is wanted, respected, and has worth is the basis of combating depression and freeing energy for living.

CONSERVATION OF STRUCTURAL INTEGRITY

Cognitive changes are caused and increased by the sensory and perceptual decline related to aging. Risk of injury increases. The environment (home or institution) must be adjusted to failing vision, hearing, and motor coordination by using brighter colors, better illumination, and supplying special telephones for the hard of hearing. Slippery floor coverings should be eliminated, and grab rails and nonskid treads installed (Butler and Lewis 1973).

When planning care for an older person, the nurse should ask whether he needs glasses or a hearing aid. Is his so-called cognitive decline perhaps a loss of sensory contact? Recent memory loss can be hazardous if the environment is not adapted or some lifelong habits are not changed — smoking in bed, cooking with long sleeves, using a kettle without a loud whistle.

When positioning, transferring, and walking with paretic patients who are confused about their body parts or function, the nurse must adapt her interventions to conserve anatomical and physiological integrity. A person who is disoriented and unsure of his own judgment often cannot describe or report pain; the nurse can only assess his pain and discomfort by observing his behavior. Another difficult task toward conserving physiological integrity is supervising a confused person's medication consumption: kind, time, and amount.

CONSERVATION OF PERSONAL INTEGRITY

Boredom, purposelessness, and *"aloneness,* or the fear for physical survival in a threatening uncertain world, . . . and *loneliness;* the fear of emotional isolation, of being locked inside oneself . . . unable to obtain warmth and comfort" all can lead to cognitive impairment (Butler and Lewis 1973). The staff's countertransference feelings, unresolved fears of aging and death — often expressed verbally and nonverbally — add to the patient's feelings of low self-worth and fearfulness.

Confusion and incontinence as tokens of failing control and utter dependency are a threat to the caretaker. Nursing means close physical contact: it is embarrassing to watch a man who could be your father expose himself. Reversing the relationship and relating to the older person as if he were a child is an attempt to quiet one's own anxiety, but to the aged person, the price is shame and lowered self-esteem.

In working with the aged, one cannot provide nursing care without working through one's own feelings toward aging, death, dependency, and perhaps the absurdity of human existence. Genuine respect and nonpossessive warmth are the basis for a relationship of trust and security, a *sine qua non* for helping a person rebuild his integrity.

Building trust implies: "You can rely on me; I shall be available; nothing detrimental that can possibly be prevented will happen to you." Trust also implies that the patient assumes some responsibility for himself, even if his abilities seem marginal. Decision-making is left to the client unless his decision will lead to hurt or shame to him or others. It is essential to work with the patient's assets at a gradual pace and respect his resistance.

Mr. N.'s care illustrates how we worked with resistance and decision-making. He was single, 50 years old, and had a responsible position and strong religious background. Mr. N. was diagnosed as having normal-pressure hydrocephalus, and a shunt was inserted. His speech was aggressive and full of sexual allusions. He pinched any nurse who dared come near. Our explicit contract was: no pinching, but all decisions about his daily routine and/or verbal expression were up to him. I tried to convey to him that my expectations were high.

For two weeks, he refused to take a bath, use a knife and fork, or go to the bathroom. Understandably, some personnel resisted what we were doing, but the contract was honored. After two weeks, he asked me to take him to the shower. He paced his return to socially acceptable norms in the presence of someone "to rely on," someone who was setting limits, nonrestricting though they were.

A confused person cannot rely upon his own testing of reality. To go along with unacceptable behavior in order to avoid upsetting him only adds to his insecurity and confusion. A consistent, repeated process of consensual validation is necessary (Sullivan 1953). Even with the very confused and deteriorated person, it is important to pick out his meaningful comments and continue talking with him (Hayter 1974). Reminders of objective reality—clocks, calendars, family photographs—are helpful, too (Burnside 1970).

Concrete symbols of one's past can offer the reassurance of continuity to the self now severely threatened by brain disease. Ms. D., aged 52, had Alzheimer's disease, a progressive deterioration of cognitive functioning. To keep herself oriented, she hung an entire wall with pictures of herself and set up what might strike a visitor as a shrine, with all the tangible achievements of her past—the books she wrote, paintings she made, correspondence with famous contemporaries. Ms. D. found her own solution, but it is often up to us to be aware of a person's past and to help turn objects into visible, touchable grabrails.

Physical and mental privacy means a great deal to an old person. Often, nurses have to provide this for him. His territoriality and material belongings must be respected (Roberts 1973).

We can listen thoughtfully to the reminiscences of a cognitively impaired person and let him find his way and meaning in life by reviewing his past. This review can help him to rebuild his personal integrity and perhaps to achieve integrity rather than despair in Erikson's sense (Butler 1968).

Learning is a principal tool in regaining and maintaining personal integrity, and it is best achieved through slow or self-paced tasks and a supportive atmosphere. Teaching the aged to organize information and to use mediators is one way to enhance learning. Mr. R. could not remember when to take which medication. We asked him about his daily meals. He reported he always had coffee for breakfast, juice with lunch, and a glass of wine after dinner. Colors were chosen as mediators. The bottles of pills he needed to take in the morning were taped brown (one pill, one stripe of tape—three pills from another bottle, three stripes). The one for lunch was taped yellow as his orange juice, and the evening medication, red as his wine. With these simple, but to him, meaningful associations, he was able to be responsible for his own medications. It was also important to augment what he learned visually by talking it over with him (Canestrari 1963; Botwinick 1973: Eisdorfer 1970). These approaches to relearning need to be adapted to the teaching of self-care, ambulation, speech and social orientation.

Simple, small pleasures—a special dish, a favorite drink, a trip, flowers, a pet, a gift—along with respect and genuine concern, add to a patient's sense of personal integrity.

CONSERVATION OF SOCIAL INTEGRITY

Every human being gains understanding of his meaning and self-worth from his interaction with others. To help conserve the patient's social integrity, the nurse must be available to the family so that they will not withdraw from the patient. She must explain what has happened to the patient, guide the family in ways they can help, and enable different members to work through feelings which range from helplessness and love to anxiety, depression, and anger.

Chronic brain syndrome severely strains interpersonal relationships within the family and community. Often a family cannot foresee what problems may arise when an elderly person leaves the hospital. The cultural stigma attached to mental and degenerative disease raises many fears and questions. Who in the community should be told? How and what should children be told about the older person? Will other relatives share the same fate? Is the condition hereditary?

Often, the family is so overwhelmed by a confused patient at home that problems become compounded. It becomes necessary for nursing staff to raise questions, focus attention, help sort out issues, suggest possible solutions, and consider what the alternatives might be (Savitsky and Sharkey 1972; Cath 1972; Berezin 1970; Soyer 1972).

Reactivation of earlier family conflicts adds to the difficulty of dealing with the present. Partial unresolved grief and helplessness are often dealt with by denial, projection, and reaction-formation. A nurse can help family members gradually face the unavoidable reality of the older member's mental decline, accept outbursts of anger and hostility, and examine guilt feelings together.

Self-sacrifice is one way some family members try to cope with an overwhelming situation. Letting individuals realize that this can harm them and other family members, as well as the patient, may ease their guilt feelings. Soyer (1972) points out:

Our purpose becomes that of helping the family cope in a way that is consistent, not with some objective sense of right or wrong, but with the family's own needs, its life patterns, its sense of worth. Whatever the "solution" it chooses, the family should be left some degree of comfort and sense of integrity, even if it must choose a course that is really not in the best interests of the older person himself.

Examining and activating the available community resources can provide some relief. Ms. B., with presenile dementia, was always a center of social action in her community. Her disoriented, bothersome behavior scared and repulsed former friends. Only after the medical nature of her disease was interpreted to the people in her close-knit community could they rally to help her and her family.

Working with the cognitively impaired aged themselves, Irene Burnside (1969, 1971, and 1973) employs resocialization, remotivation, reality orientation, touch, and the life review. A major goal in her group work with the institutionalized aged is to rebuild their social integrity.

Nursing care that leads to optimal conservation of poor assets can make a difference to the individual and the family disturbed by events as devastating as a mental impairment.

REFERENCES

Agate, J.: Special Hazards of Illness in Later Life, in Rossman, I., et al. (eds.): *Clinical Geriatrics* (Philadelphia: J. B. Lippincott Co., 1971).

Berezin, M.: Partial grief in family members and others who care for the elderly patient, J. Geriatr. Psychiatry 4:53, 1970.

128   MIRIAM J. HIRSCHFELD

Botwinick, J.: *Aging and Behavior* (New York: Springer Publishing Co., 1973)

Burnside, I. M.: Group work among the aged, Nurs. Outlook 17:68, 1969.

Burnside, I. M.: Clocks and calendars, Am. J. Nurs. 70:117, 1970.

Burnside, I. M.: Long term group work with hospitalized aged, Gerontologist 11 (3):213, 1971.

Burnside, I. M. (ed.): *Psychosocial Nursing Care of the Aged* (New York: McGraw-Hill Book Co., 1973).

Butler, R.: The Life Review: An Interpretation of Reminiscence in the Aged, in Neugarten, B. (ed.): *Middle Age and Aging* (Chicago: The University of Chicago Press, 1968), pp. 486–496.

Butler, R. N., and Lewin, M. I.: *Aging and Mental Health* (St. Louis: C. V. Mosby Company, 1973).

Canestrari, R. E.: Paced and self-paced learning in young and elderly adults, J. Gerontol. 18:165, 1963.

Cath, S. H.: The institutionalization of a parent—a nadir of life, J. Geriatr. Psychiatry 5:25, 1972.

Eisdorfer, C.: Intellectual and Cognitive Changes in the Aged, in Busse, E. W., and Pfeiffer, E. (eds.): *Behavior and Adaptation in Late Life* (Boston: Little, Brown and Co., 1970), pp. 237–250.

Hayter, J.: Patients who have Alzheimer's disease, Am. J. Nurs. 74:1460, 1974.

Kahn, R.: Psychological Aspects of Aging, in Rossman, I., et al. (eds.): *Clinical Geriatrics* (Philadelphia: J. B. Lippincott Co., 1971), pp. 107–114.

Levine, M. E.: *Introduction to Clinical Nursing* (Philadelphia: F. A. Davis, 1973).

Lindemann, E.: Symptomatology and Management of Acute Grief, in Parad, H. J. (ed.): *Crisis Intervention: Selected Readings* (New York: Family Service Association of America, 1965), pp. 7–21.

Roberts, S. L.: Territoriality: Space and the Aged Patient in Intensive Care Units, in Burnside, I. M. (ed.): *Psychosocial Nursing Care of the Aged* (New York: McGraw-Hill Book Co., 1973), pp. 72–83.

Savitsky, E., and Sharkey, H.: Study of family interaction in the aged, J. Geriatr. Psychiatry 5:3, 1972.

Soyer, D.: Helping the family to live with itself, J. Geriatr. Psychiatry 5:52, 1972.

Sullivan, H. S.: *The Interpersonal Theory of Psychiatry* (New York: W. W. Norton and Co., 1953).

Wang, H. S.: Organic Brain Syndromes, in Busse, E. W., and Pfeiffer, E. (eds.): *Behavior and Adaptation in Late Life* (Boston: Little, Brown and Co., 1970), pp. 263–288.

10 / The Use of Medication to Prevent Custodial Care

HEINZ E. LEHMANN, M.D.
Director of Medical Education and Research, Douglas Hospital, and Professor of Psychiatry, McGill University, Montreal, Quebec, Canada.

THERE EXISTS for the aged, in response to various life stresses, a well-known vicious psychosomatic pattern that may be represented as follows. Life events can lead to persistent negative affective response, which is the same as stress. Stress can lead to disturbed balance of neuroendocrine factors (norepinephrine; serotonin). This results in impaired metabolic functioning of cerebral tissue, which in turn causes reduced metabolic demands of brain tissue, resulting in decreased blood flow to the brain which leads to relative cerebral ischemia, cerebral hypoxia and irreversible loss of vulnerable neurons. This loss results in further loss of mental capacity, causing further persistent negative affective response and further stress. The pattern progresses in a downward spiral.

Until the stage of neuronal loss is reached, toward the end of this destructive process, some interventions, either psychosocial or psychopharmacologic in nature, are possible and may partly halt or even reverse the process. The psychopharmacologic or medication approach can influence this vicious cycle and, to some extent, may help prevent or reduce the need of custodial care for the aged.

The best environment for an aged person — with few exceptions — is his own household, with his family, or living alone. The factors that determine whether an old person lives with his family or alone are usually beyond therapeutic reach because they are of a social-existential nature, e.g., death of spouse, physical absence of children, individual preferences. But whether living in a family setting or alone, the elderly person preserves his autonomy. He may be robbed of it, how-

129

ever, by pathological factors, i.e., either physical illness or mental disabilities or far-advanced senescence.

Custodial care is an alternative for those unable to maintain a family or autonomous life in the community. One may conceive of custodial care as care given within an institutional setting. In this sense, the varieties of custodial care can be ranked according to the loss of autonomy they imply and thus to their desirability, ranging from an old people's home to nursing home to hospital. Between any of these stages, an increase of pathology determines the transition. At any of these transitional points either psychosocial or pharmacologic interventions may be possible.

The most important task for psychosocial or drug interventions, then, is prophylactic in nature: the prevention of the development of pathology that is severe enough to change the elderly person's status from independence to dependence on custodial care. In regard to psychosocial interventions, a limited preventative impact may be ascribed to such factors as keeping an aging individual active, emotionally involved, and exposed to as many interpersonal contacts as possible.

Pharmacologic prevention of the development of pathology aims at the relatively healthy elderly person who as yet shows no, or only insignificant, signs and symptoms of the disability of old age. A high priority for future efforts is to alert the public to become concerned about possible physical, emotional, and cognitive deficiencies of aging long before they are clearly noticeable.

Unfortunately we have at present no drugs that are known to reliably prevent or reduce the disabilities of normal aging—even less the ravages of arteriosclerosis or senile dementia. Research effort should be aimed at developing pharmacologic aids that will be capable of preventing the disabilities of old age. Meanwhile there are situations where medication can alleviate symptoms that might lead to a decision for custodial care.

REASONS FOR CUSTODIAL CARE

The most important factors contributing to the decision to arrange for custodial care of an aged person are: extreme agitation, accompanied by insomnia and, frequently, by irritability and aggressiveness; serious danger of accidents caused by confusion, e.g., unintentionally causing a fire or wandering away and getting lost; special treatment problems, e.g., fractures or incontinence in an elderly, overweight person. Other reasons for custodial care exist either if the old person is too stressful for the family, particularly if he is demanding and crotchety; or if the family is too stressful for the old person, e.g., if there are many noisy children, if the quarters are too crowded, or if there are intolerant in-laws.

The advantages of custodial care should not be overlooked. They include the continuous supervision that can be provided and the special facilities for care and treatment that are available in a hospital setting, i.e., trained medical and paramedical staff, special toileting and bedcare equipment, and facilities for treatment such as intravenous infusions, occupational therapy, and physiotherapy. Finally, another advantage of institutional care for an old person is the relief that the family enjoys when freed from the responsibility and the inconveniences that are connected with the care of the elderly.

The disadvantages of institutional, custodial care include the trauma of displacement and rejection to which the aged person is subjected when he is sent away and the inconveniences for him of having to adjust to new routines, to a new diet, and to certain restrictions of his freedom. Other disadvantages are the difficulties of finding adequate accommodation in a home or a hospital bed and the not inconsiderable cost of institutional care. Finally, the risk of developing institutionalism, i.e., loss of motivation, initiative, independence, and vitality, is always present and often unavoidable when an aged person is placed in custodial care.

On the other side, the advantages of looking after an elderly person in the family, even if he is slightly or moderately disabled, are that the setting is more therapeutic and therefore more likely to restore a person with impaired functioning to his former level of performance or to prevent or delay the development of further impairment, as well as that the aged person has a better chance in a family setting to avoid chronicity and to learn how to cope with his disabilities. Last, but not least, the often intense guilt that family members may feel when they place an aged relative into an old people's home, a nursing home, or a hospital is avoided.

PSYCHOTROPIC DRUGS FOR GEROPSYCHIATRIC SYMPTOMS

The main psychiatric symptoms that are often responsible for transferring a patient from independent to dependent care are insomnia, agitation, irritability and aggression, depression, psychotic symptoms, lethargy, and confusion. These symptoms are often treatable with drugs (Table 10–1).

Insomnia.—As a rule, sleep disturbances respond well to the vari-

TABLE 10-1.—PSYCHOTROPIC DRUGS
FOR GEROPSYCHIATRIC SYMPTOMS

SYMPTOM	MEDICATION
Insomnia	Hypnotics
Agitation	Major and minor tranquilizers
Irritability	Major and minor tranquilizers
Depression	Antidepressants
Psychotic symptoms	Major tranquilizers
Lethargy	Psychostimulants
Confusion	Nootropic drugs

ous hypnotic drugs on the market. It is generally recommended that barbiturates not be prescribed for geriatric patients, because they may cause "paradoxical" effects and excite the patient by producing disinhibition. This is by no means always so, and there are many geriatric patients who respond well to appropriate doses of barbiturates. However, there are less toxic hypnotic drugs than barbiturates today—not methyprylon (Noludar), glutethimide (Doriden) or ethchlorvynol (Placidyl) or methaqualone (Quaalude), which are just as toxic—but the benzodiazepines, e.g., flurazepam (Dalmane), or diazepam (Valium) in doses twice those used for daytime sedation. The sedative phenothiazines, e.g., chlorpromazine (Largactil; Thorazine) or thioridazine (Mellaril), also have excellent hypnotic properties, particularly when prescribed in staggered, increasing doses, e.g., 10 mg of thioridazine at 3 P.M., 25 mg at 6 P.M., and 50–75 mg at 8 P.M. To counteract the tendency of geriatric patients to slow absorption, and in order to avoid delayed effects of the drugs that would leave the patient restless at night and drowsy the next day, it is advisable to give hypnotic drugs fairly early in the evening and with a hot beverage. Very small doses of a tricyclic antidepressant, e.g., 3–5 mg of amitriptyline added to the nighttime sedative often prolong its action and allow the patient to sleep longer in the morning.

Confusion might be increased by hypnotics; this is least likely to occur with phenothiazines. Since nocturnal restlessness, unresponsive to casual sedation, is a frequent reason for wanting to transfer a patient from his home to an institution or from an institutional home to a hospital, it is important to work out an individual, effective nighttime prescription for each patient within the first two or three days after the issue has become critical.

Agitation, irritability, aggression.—Agitation and irritability are threatening to the people caring for the elderly and are among the most common reasons given for wanting to transfer a geropsychiatric patient. Yet, both symptoms respond specifically to psychotropic medication. If the agitation is associated primarily with anxiety, the antianxiety medications are most effective; if aggression prevails, the antipsychotics (neuroleptics) are often a better choice. Dosage, as well as time and frequency of administration, are critical factors in geriatric patients. Drugs indicated for daytime sedation include meprobamate; or a benzodiazepine, e.g., chlordiazepoxide (Librium); or diazepam (Valium); some antihistaminics, e.g., diphenhydramine (Benadryl); sedative phenothiazines, e.g., chlorpromazine or thioridazine; or a thioxanthene, e.g., chlorprothixene (Taractan).

It is always advisable to start with small doses in geriatric patients, i.e., one quarter or one half the usual adult dose, and then gradually, sometimes more rapidly, to increase the dose until the effective dose has been reached. Since the pharmacologic action of the drugs after parenteral administration becomes apparent within 20–30 minutes, another dose should be administered about 30–40 minutes after the first injection if the patient is still excited. After oral administration, the effects of tranquilizers may be delayed for 1 hour or 2. At any rate, it is important *not* to wait until the effects of the first dose have completely disappeared before giving the next one. Hypotension and extrapyramidal symptoms are troublesome side effects, particularly of the antipsychotic medications (neuroleptics). Hypotension is less likely to develop in agitated patients, and extrapyramidal symptoms appear, as a rule, only after a week or two of continuous administration, and not when the drugs are only used for symptomatic sedation for a limited time.

Depression.—Depression is the most common functional psychiatric syndrome in geriatric patients, and the incidence of suicide increases with age. Depressed old patients often manifest symptoms of an organic brain syndrome (pseudodementia), e.g., confusion and cognitive disorders, that may disappear completely once the depression has cleared up. Geriatric patients, in general, respond well to tricyclic antidepressants. The use of MAO inhibitors in the elderly is not advisable, except in the hospital, because of the many interactions of these drugs with other medications, various food items, and alcohol. A depressed old person may not be able to remember all the things he is supposed to avoid in his diet and medications.

The effective dose for most tricyclic antidepressants, e.g., imipramine (Tofranil) or amitriptyline (Elavil), is 100–200 mg per day, most or all of which should be given at bedtime. However, many geriatric patients are overly sensitive to the anticholinergic, hypotensive, and sedative effects of these drugs, and will have to be treated with much smaller doses. Doxepin (Sinequan) is, in our experience, particularly well tolerated by geriatric patients. In any case, one should always start with small doses in geriatric patients and then gradually increase the dosage as the patient's tolerance to the drug is established. Confusional toxic states may be induced in susceptible geriatric patients, even with small doses of tricyclic antidepressants. We have seen an old lady, 82 years of age, become acutely confused and develop visual hallucinations after 3 days of treatment with only 30 mg of amitriptyline per day; she recovered from this state 2 days after the antidepressant was discontinued.

In view of the considerable risk of suicide and the generally favorable results with antidepressant therapy in depressed geriatric patients, a carefully prescribed and monitored trial with tricyclic antidepressants for at least 4–6 weeks is always indicated for depression. An awareness of the possible cardiotoxic effects of the tricyclic antidepressants is a consideration when prescribing to older patients and could be a contraindication in some individuals.

Psychotic symptoms.—The antipsychotic drugs (neuroleptics) are specifically effective in suppressing psychotic symptoms, such as hallucinations, delusions, and thought disorder. Anticholinergic and other side effects affecting the autonomic nervous system are most frequently observed with aliphatic (e.g., chlorpromazine) and piperidine (e.g., thioridazine) derivatives of phenothiazine. These derivatives also have the most sedating effects, at least for the first week or two, until tolerance to these effects has been developed. The piperazine derivatives of phenothiazine, the thioxanthene, thiothixene (Navane), and the butyrophenones produce fewer autonomic and sedative but more extrapyramidal side effects. Geropsychiatric.patients are particularly sensitive to the piperazine derivatives, thiothixene and the butyrophenones, and they are also at greater risk to develop the dreaded complication of irreversible tardive dyskinesia. On the other hand, cerebral circulation in geriatric patients is easily compromised by drug-induced hypotension. This means that the clinician has to steer a judicious and careful course when treating psychotic symptoms in geriatric patients—between trying to avoid the Scylla of hypotension and the Charybdis of extrapyramidal complications in his choice of antipsychotic drugs (major tranquilizers, neuroleptics). As with many other medications in geriatric patients, the doses should be kept at one half or one quarter of the usual adult dose, at least at the beginning of pharmacotherapy, and then gradually increased to their optimal level.

Psychotic symptoms, e.g., paranoid delusions which develop so commonly in geriatric patients, can be very frightening to the people in the family or in the nursing home who care for these patients, and are often the reason for their transfer. On the other hand, the therapeutic results with antipsychotic drugs in these conditions are often very gratifying, regardless of the age of the patients.

Lethargy. — Inertia, lethargy, and apathy are difficult to combat with medication in geriatric patients. The obvious drugs for this condition, the psychostimulants like dextroamphetamine (Dexedrine), methylphenidate (Ritalin), pentylenetetrazol (Metrazol), and caffeine are only of limited value. The amphetamine-like drugs with adrenergic activity easily overshoot their mark, and instead of increased initiative and motivation they often produce excessive tension, anxiety, restlessness, and insomnia. In addition, these drugs tend to aggravate existing psychotic symptoms, such as delusions and hallucinations, and may even evoke them in patients who did not manifest them before.

Pentylenetetrazol has been shown in a few controlled studies to bring about improvement of some symptoms in geropsychiatric patients, but the results that can be obtained with it are far from spectacular (Prien 1973; Lehmann and Ban 1974). Caffeine has not been studied systematically for its effects in geropsychiatric patients, but general clinical experience has shown that it is useful as a mild stimulant that does not increase confusion or aggravate psychotic symptoms.

Confusion. — Confusion may be considered to be a core symptom of both the acute and chronic organic brain syndrome. Its incidence is high in geriatric patients, and a confused patient can become very troublesome for the personnel caring for him. Thus, confusion is often the reason given for transferring a geropsychiatric patient from one facility to another.

We know at this time no drug whose activity is specifically directed at the correction of confusional states. However, a new class of psychotropic drugs has recently been introduced by the Belgian pharmacologist Giurgea (1973), who proposed to call it the class of *nootropic* drugs.

NOOTROPIC DRUGS

The drug which Giurgea studied, and on which he based his concept of nootropic substances is piracetam, a GABA (gamma-aminobutyric acid) derivative. In animal experiments this drug acts selectively on telencephalic integrative mechanisms, promotes interhemispheric transfer, protects against experimental amnesic agents, and facilitates electroencephalographic recovery after severe hypoxia (Sara and Lefevre 1972). The drug has virtually no effects on autonomic functions, arousal level, limbic lobe activity, or psychomotor behavior. In controlled clinical trials with geropsychiatric patients and elderly persons with subclinical symptoms of senescence, this drug produced significant improvement of behavior and improvement in the performance of mental tasks demanding vigilance and acuity, with no side effects whatsoever (Steglink 1972; Mindus et al. 1975). Although piracetam cannot reverse marked mental deterioration and is effective only in states of mild cerebral insufficiency, its selective action on telencephalic structures, and the absence of toxicity and side effects make it an extremely interesting representative of the new nootropic class of psychoactive drugs.

Other substances that were developed during the last decade and that have been successfully tried in the management of senile and senescent symptoms, as well as in the treatment of acute confusional states, have been shown in animals to reduce the accumulation of the age pigment lipofuscin; to increase cerebral glucose metabolism; to improve cerebral circulation; or to improve cellular metabolism in the brain through modification of essential enzyme activity. They are: centrophenoxim (Espie 1966; Coirault et al. 1962), Hydergine (Cerletti et al. 1973; Bazo 1973), and naftidrofuryl (Judge and Urquhart 1972; Bouvier et al. 1974).

None of these drugs have been studied sufficiently to be certain that their properties would match the requirements for a truly nootropic—"mind acting"—drug; i.e., selective telencephalic action with few primary effects on autonomic, emotional, and arousal functions. Nevertheless, a new perspective has been opened in that direction, and promising research is going on in this area.

In conclusion, custodial care of the geropsychiatric patient should be avoided or delayed by all available psychosocial measures, and these measures should be supplemented by psychotropic medication. The psychiatric and behavioral problems that are usually responsible for transferring an elderly person from his home to custodial care can be identified, and many of them can be specifically and effectively counteracted by well-chosen medication. Dosage and side effects cause more problems in geropsychiatric patients than in younger adults, but with carefully chosen individual prescriptions and continued monitoring of the patient's condition, many elderly people can be spared the trauma of institutionalization and can be protected against the possible damages of custodial care.

REFERENCES

Bazo, A. J.: An ergot alkaloid preparation (hydergine) versus papaverine in treating common complaints of the aged: Double-blind study, J. Am. Geriatr. Soc. 21:63, 1973.

Becker, K., and Hoyer, S.: Studies on cerebral metabolism during pyrithioxine treatment, Dtsch Z. Nervenheilk. 188:200, 1966.

Bouvier, J. B., Passeron, O., and Chupin, M. P.: Psychometric study on Praxilene, J. Int. Med. Res. 2:59, 1974.

Cerletti, A., Emmenegger, H., Meier-Ruge, W., et al.: Experimental Cerebral Insufficiency. Models for the Quantification of Dihydrogenated Ergot Effects on Brain Metabolism and Function. Scientific exhibit, Federation of American Societies for Experimental Biology, 57th Annual Meeting, April 15–20, 1973, Atlantic City, N. J.

Coirault, R., Jarret, T., Ramel, P., Cadour, E., Crocq, L., and Vincent, A.: Dimethyl-amino-ethyl ester of parachlorophenoxy acetic acid – its psychopathological action, J. Neuropsychiat. 3:367, 1962.

Espie, J.: Pharmacologie de la centrophénoxine. Application au delirium tremens, Lyon Med. 215:935, 1966.

Giurgea, C.: The "nootropic" approach to the integrative activity of the brain, Cond. Reflex 8:108, 1973.

Hadlik, J., Sindelarova, M., and Svestka, J.: Experimental and clinical experience with Encephabol therapy in geropsychiatry, Cesk. Psychiatr. 67:129, 1971.

Judge, T. G., and Urquhart, Anne: Naftidrofuryl – a double-blind cross-over study in the elderly, Curr. Med. Res. Opin. 1:166, 1972.

Lehmann, H. E., and Ban, T. A.: Psychological tests: Practice effect in geriatric patients, Geriatrics 23:160, 1968.

Lehmann, H. E., and Ban, T. A.: Psychometric tests in evaluation of brain pathology, response to drugs, Geriatrics 25:142, 1970.

Lehmann, H. E., and Ban, T. A.: Central Nervous System Stimulants and Anabolic Substances in Geropsychiatric Therapy, in Gershon, S., and Raskin, A. (eds.): *Aging*, vol. 2 (New York: Raven Press, 1975), pp. 179–202.

Mindus, P., Cronholm, B., Levander, S. E., and Schalling, D.: Piracetam and Mental Performance in Aging People. Presented at the APA Annual Meeting, May 5–9, 1975, Anaheim, Calif.

Prien, R. F.: *Chronic Organic Brain Syndrome. A Review of the Therapeutic*

Literature with Special Emphasis on Chemotherapy (Washington, D.C.: Veterans Administration, Dept. of Medicine and Surgery, 1972).

Sara, S. J., and Lefevre, D.: Hypoxia-induced amnesia in one-trial learning and pharmacological protection by piracetam, Psychopharmacologia 25:32, 1972.

Stegink, A. J.: The clinical use of piracetam, a new nootropic drug: The treatment of symptoms of senile involution, Arzneim. Forsch. 22:975, 1972.

11/ Pharmacokinetics of Psychotherapeutic Agents in Aged Patients

ROBERT O. FRIEDEL, M.D.
Associate Professor and Vice Chairman, Department of Psychiatry and Behavioral Sciences, University of Washington, Seattle, Washington

THE TREATMENT of the elderly patient with senile dementia or other mental disorders frequently involves the use of a variety of medications, as outlined in the preceding chapter by Doctor Lehmann. However, the use of pharmacologic agents in treating older patients presents special problems, since the aged typically show greater variation in response to drugs than the young (Friedel and Raskind 1977). This altered response pattern may be due to age-dependent changes in tissue sensitivity to drugs as well as in their *absorption, distribution, metabolism* and *excretion*. It is the purpose of this chapter to discuss the effects of alterations in these last four factors, referred to as *pharmacokinetic processes*, on drug response in the elderly. These processes are important because they influence the concentration of drugs in the blood and this, in turn, determines their concentration in target organs. For drugs which are known to bind reversibly with their receptor sites — and these constitute the great majority of psychotherapeutic agents — the concentration of the drug in the biosphere of the receptor is felt to determine the degree of effect. In contrast, the blood levels of such drugs as reserpine and monoamine oxidase inhibitors, which bind irreversibly to their receptors, do not accurately reflect the intensity of pharmacologic activity.

In patients receiving identical doses of psychotherapeutic agents, the differences in plasma concentrations are considerable, often greater than 20-fold at the two extremes. In addition to a discussion of some of the factors which may cause these marked differences in blood levels (and therefore differences in clinical effect) in the aged patient, recent data reflecting upon the clinical utility of determining blood levels of one such drug in a population of elderly patients with depression will also be presented.

Before proceeding to an analysis of the factors involved in pharmacokinetics, however, it may be helpful to consider the quantitative relationship of several of those factors to drug blood concentration (Greenblatt and Koch-Weser 1975). The following equation represents this relationship under those circumstances most commonly encountered in clinical practice, i.e., a fixed dose of drug given at specific time intervals:

$$\overline{C}_\infty = 1.44 \times \frac{fD \times t_{1/2\beta}}{V_d \times \tau}$$

where $\overline{C}_\infty$ represents the average steady-state concentration of the drug in the blood, fD is the absorbed dose, $t_{1/2\beta}$ is the elimination half-life, V_d is the apparent volume of the distribution of drug in the body, and τ is the dosage interval. It is apparent from this equation, as well as intuitively reasonable, that the steady-state blood level of a drug is directly proportional to the amount of drug absorbed and to the time it takes to eliminate the drug from the body, while inversely related to the volume in which the drug is distributed and to the time between doses of the same quantity. Although it is not apparent from this equation, for most drugs given at a dosage interval less than or equal to the elimination half-life, the steady-state concentration at that dose will be achieved in approximately 5 half-lives. It is important to understand this last observation and to **avoid** raising drug dosage so rapidly that the therapeutic range is exceeded and toxic levels are reached because of drug accumulation.

ABSORPTION

Absorption of drugs is defined quantitatively in terms of *bioavailability*, a term used to indicate the amount of drug which reaches the general circulation and the rate at which it does so. Both factors, quantity and rate, are important since together they influence the eventual blood level which a drug reaches following a single dose. For drugs administered on a fixed schedule, the rate of absorption becomes less important than the fraction of the dose absorbed, since accumulation will occur as long as the dosage interval is short enough. The biological effect, it is to be remembered, depends upon reaching at least the minimal effective concentration of the agent in question.

Biological membranes are permeable to water, small lipid insoluble substances, and lipid soluble substances. Since, with the exception of lithium, most psychotherapeutic agents are not small molecules, their absorption is governed largely by their lipid solubility. Lipid solubility in turn depends upon the degree of ionization of the drug, since nonionized molecules are more lipid soluble. Ionization, in turn, depends on the pK of the molecule and the pH of the medium. Weak organic acids, such as the barbiturates, will be less ionized and more readily absorbed at the acidic pH of the stomach, while weak bases, such as the tricyclic antidepressants, will be less ionized in the small intestine where the pH of the intestinal contents is approximately 6.6.

Many other factors affect the absorption of drugs, including the route of administration, stomach contents, and the degree of gut and liver metabolism. While a variety of psychotherapeutic agents reach the general circulation more efficiently following parenteral administration, this cannot always be assumed to be the case. Chlordiazepoxide (Greenblatt et al. 1974) and diazepam (Hillestad 1974), for example, are absorbed less well after intramuscular injection than after oral administration. It is felt that these drugs crystallize at the site of IM injection, thereby decreasing their bioavailability. Presystemic metabolism of drugs, such as chlorpromazine, may occur in the gut wall by saturable enzyme systems (Hollister et al. 1970). Therefore, given the same quantity of medication per day, frequent small doses of drugs so metabolized may result in a lower steady-state drug blood level than larger doses given less often. A smaller fraction of the medication will be metabolized when larger doses are given less often.

Since the liver is the major site of drug metabolism in the body, the amount of liver metabolism which occurs following absorption of the drug from the GI tract into the portal system (referred to as the *first-pass effect*) will significantly influence the fraction of the dose reaching the general circulation. Alterations in liver blood flow and the liver's ability to metabolize the drug, therefore, may result in marked changes in bioavailability (Wilkinson and Shand 1975).

Theoretically, it is possible then for all of these factors to cause age-related changes in drug absorption in either direction. Few pharmacokinetic studies have been performed to evaluate the effects of age on the absorption of psychotherapeutic agents. Absorption of orally administered diazepam (Garattini et al. 1973) and chlordiazepoxide

(Shader et al. 1977) are decreased in the elderly, but it should not be assumed that this is the case for all drugs.

DISTRIBUTION

The second factor affecting drug blood levels is distribution, quantitatively expressed as apparent volume of distribution (V_d). The intravascular space in the average adult is 3–4 liters; the extracellular space is approximately 12 liters; and the total body water is about 41 liters. If all drugs were distributed homogenously through the total body water, the apparent volume of distribution would be 41 liters and a single compartment model of drug distribution would be adequate. Most psychotherapeutic agents, however, are not distributed homogenously throughout the body. Many of these drugs are selectively concentrated in certain tissues such as brain, liver, red blood cells, fat, or other tissues. Consequently, a single compartment model is too simplistic, and a multiple compartment model must be employed to more closely represent the physiological state. The most frequently used is the two-compartment open model in which it is assumed that absorption and elimination of the drug takes place rapidly into and from a small central compartment consisting of the blood and the extracellular fluid of rapidly perfused tissues. From this central compartment the drug slowly enters and leaves a larger peripheral compartment consisting of tissues less well perfused. The relative volume of these compartments varies from one drug to another and depends upon the affinity of particular drugs for the tissues involved. It is apparent from the blood drug concentration equation that at a given absorbed dose, half-life, and dosage interval, the greater the apparent volume into which a particular drug is distributed, the lower the steady-state blood level, and, therefore, the lower the concentration of the drug in the target tissue.

Since most psychotherapeutic agents are lipid soluble, they have a significant affinity for fat tissue. With aging, the adipose tissue-lean tissue ratio typically increases (Lasagna 1956; Korenchevsky 1961; Gregerman and Bierman 1974), and therefore the volume of distribution of lipid soluble drugs in the elderly patient is usually greater than in younger people of the same size. Indeed, this has been shown to be the case for diazepam (Klotz et al. 1975). The age-related decreases in the volumes of distribution of thyroxine (Gregerman et al. 1962) and propicillin (Simon et al. 1972), which are more soluble than diazepam, and therefore probably distributed differently in body tissues, may also be related to adipose tissue-lean tissue body mass.

There are two other important factors to be remembered regarding drug distribution in the body. The first factor is that the unbound plasma drug concentration is in equilibrium with the target tissue. Many of the psychotherapeutic agents bind extensively to serum albumin and red blood cells. For example, the tricyclic antidepressants are bound in the range of 80–95% to plasma proteins (Glassman et al. 1973); this leaves only the remaining 5–20% for activity. Differences in drug binding are related to genetic factors, a variety of disease states such as hypoalbuminemia, or the administration of drugs (such as salicylates) which displace other drugs from these sites. The second additional factor, as previously noted, is that penetration of cell membranes by large organic molecules depends upon their lipid solubility. Thus, the blood brain barrier is readily crossed by physostigmine, a tertiary amine used in the treatment of CNS toxic reactions caused by anticholinergic agents such as tricyclic antidepressants and antiparkinson agents. Neostigmine, while an equally effective cholinesterase inhibitor, is a quaternary amine and, therefore, does not readily enter the CNS.

METABOLISM

Differences in the metabolism of psychotherapeutic agents in the liver and other tissues may also explain variation in drug response. The relative rates of conversion of a drug to its active and/or inactive metabolites and the effects of other drugs or substances on the enzymatic processes involved may vary substantially from one patient to another, resulting in marked differences in the effective life of the drug (see the drug blood concentration equation). Demethylation, oxidation, and hydroxylation appear to be the major metabolic conversions for most psychotherapeutic agents. Recent work suggests that an understanding of the relative concentrations of the parent compound and the metabolites produced by these reactions may be important in predicting a patient's response to these agents.

In the case of amphetamine, the deaminated metabolites are inactive but the hydroxy metabolite produced in the liver then enters the brain and is hydroxylated by dopamine β-hydroxylase to para-hydroxynorephedrine. This false neurotransmitter displaces norepinephrine from synaptic vesicles and results in a decrease in CNS noradrenergic activity. Differences in the relative rates of metabolism of these various pathways may explain why some patients become depressed after chronic treatment with amphetamine and others do not (Oates and Shand 1973).

The metabolism of diazepam can also proceed in several directions. First, diazepam may be demethylated to desmethyldiazepam, a metabolite which is also psychoactive. Desmethyldiazepam is then hydroxylated to another active metabolite, oxazepam. The glucuronide conjugates of hydroxy derivatives of diazepam are quite polar—therefore inactive—and are readily excreted by the kidneys. Again, the relative rates of metabolism of diazepam along these different pathways will determine the effects of this compound in a given patient.

Chlorpromazine (CPZ) can undergo many different metabolic alterations, some of them leading to inactive metabolites (CPZ-sulfoxide) and some of them leading to metabolites which are thought to be active (demethyl-CPZ, didemethyl-CPZ, hydroxy-CPZ). The tricyclic antidepressants are also demethylated to active metabolites. However, it is thought that their hydroxy metabolites are inactive. The glucuronide conjugate, of course, is inactive and readily excreted by the kidneys.

In general, there are many factors which affect drug metabolism, the most important of which is genetic. Other drugs, such as the barbiturates, caffeine, and tobacco affect drug metabolism by the induction of liver enzyme systems. Chloramphenicol, isoniazid, diphenylhydantoin, and disulfiram inhibit liver enzyme systems, thereby decreasing the metabolism of other drugs. Aging and a variety of disease states may also complicate normal drug metabolism. More specifically, the metabolism of aminopyrine (Jori et al. 1972), amobarbital (Irvine et al. 1974), and propranolol (Castleden et al. 1975) have been reported to decrease with age. These effects may be due to decrease in liver function since sodium sulfobromophthalein excretion has been shown to become increasingly impaired over the age of 50 (Thompson and Williams 1965) and the activity of liver microsomal drug-metabolizing enzymes has been shown in rats to decrease with age (Kato et al. 1964; Kato and Takanaka 1968), suggesting that a similar condition may exist in humans. Further evaluation of the contribution of age-related alterations in drug metabolism in patients not responding or responding adversely to psychotherapeutic agents will depend on the determinations of levels of the parent compound and important metabolites in the patient's blood.

EXCRETION

The elimination of most psychotherapeutic agents from the body depends essentially on two processes: (1) conversion of these lipid soluble substances to water soluble compounds (usually in the form of glucuronide or sulfate conjugate) and (2) excretion by the kidneys or other organs. The increased half-life of a drug or metabolite in any patient, or population of patients, may result from a decrease in function of either of these processes or a combination of both. The possibility of decreased metabolism of certain drugs in the aged has already been discussed. Age-related decreases in glomerular filtration, renal blood flow, and tubular excretory capacity have also been described (Goldring et al. 1940; Davies and Shock 1950; Watkin and Shock 1955; Leikola and Vartia 1957; Vartia and Leikola 1960). Digoxin and creatinine clearance in the aged have also been reported to be reduced (Ewy et al. 1969; Baylis et al. 1972), although it should be noted that the impaired ability of the kidneys in aged patients to excrete drugs is not necessarily detectable by serum creatinine determinations (Mølholm Hansen et al. 1970; Siersback-Nielsen et al. 1971). As opposed to propranolol, in which blood level elevations with aging are probably due to decreased metabolism, elevations of digoxin (Ewy et al. 1969) and practolol (Castleden et al. 1975) blood levels in the elderly have been attributed to reduction in renal function.

CLINICAL APPLICATION

The following is an example of the clinical utility of determining blood levels of psychotherapeutic agents in elderly patients. This work is being done in collaboration with Raskind at the University of Washington (Friedel and Raskind 1975). Raskind directs a geriatric outreach program in Seattle evaluating elderly patients in nursing homes and in their own homes. After a complete medical and psychiatric examination, patients are selected for treatment who meet the criteria of Feighner et al (1972) for primary or secondary affective disorder, i.e., depressed mood of at least one month's duration and at least four of the following criteria: (1) poor appetite or weight loss, (2) sleep difficulty, (3) loss of energy, (4) agitation or retardation, (5) loss of interest in usual activities or decrease in sexual drive, (6) feelings of self-reproach or guilt, (7) decreased concentration, (8) recurrent thoughts of suicide.

After the initial diagnosis is made and a clinical global impression is determined by the evaluating psychiatrist, treatment is initiated with a single dose of 50 mg of doxepin, a tricyclic antidepressant, at bedtime. The dose is increased by about 50 mg per week, until a significant response is achieved or until the treating psychiatrist is concerned about producing toxic reactions in these older, frequently more sensitive, patients. Clinical global impressions are also completed weekly, at which time blood is taken for assay 10 to 12 hours after the bedtime dose. Doxepin and its demethylated metabolite are assayed by mass fragmentography, the most selective and among the most sensitive analytical methods currently in use (Jenkins and Friedel in press). Since the metabolite is most likely also psychoactive, results are expressed as the concentration of doxepin plus desmethyldoxepin in ng/ml of plasma (Table 11–1).

Seven patients had no response or were minimally improved after treatment. The mean daily dose for this group was 104 mg, and the mean plasma concentration was 50 ng/ml. Three of these patients, treated early in the study, received only 50 mg of doxepin per day because of our concern at that time of causing serious side effects at higher levels. Eight patients demonstrated a moderate-to-marked

TABLE 11–1.—DOXEPIN PLUS DESMETHYLDOXEPIN
PLASMA LEVELS AND CLINICAL RESPONSE IN AGED
PATIENTS WITH DEPRESSION[*]

PATIENT	AGE	DAILY DOSE (MG)	PLASMA CONC. (NG/ML)	CLINICAL RESPONSE
1. F	82	50	36	Worse
2. F	65	50	45	No change
3. F	79	50	24	Minimal
4. F	67	100	48	Minimal
5. F	67	150	47	Minimal
6. F	67	250	118	No change
7. F	88	75	104	No change
		$\bar{x} = 104$	$\bar{x} = 60$	
8. F	60	150	90	Moderate
9. F	65	150	131	Marked
10. M	79	100	113	Marked
11. F	65	150	53	Moderate
12. M[†]	84	50	9	Marked
13. M	68	150	124	Moderate
14. M	63	100	138	Marked
15. F	67	300	129	Marked
		$\bar{x} = 157$	$\bar{x} = 111$	

[*]From Friedel and Raskind 1975.
[†]Not included in calculations of mean values ($\bar{x}$).

improvement of symptoms with treatment. The mean daily dose of doxepin in this group was 157 mg, and the mean plasma concentration was 111 ng/ml, the latter value differing significantly from that of the non-responder group (p < 0.015). No significant side effects were noted in any of these patients. These preliminary results suggest that a therapeutic response to doxepin in many older, depressed patients can be readily and safely achieved if blood levels are carefully monitored and if a minimum plasma level of doxepin plus desmethyldoxepin of approximately 110 ng/ml is reached. These results also demonstrate the value of performing drug and metabolite blood levels in this older patient population in order to increase the rate of therapeutic response and to decrease the incidence of toxic effects.

In summary, pharmacokinetics involves an understanding of drug absorption, distribution, metabolism, and elimination. The interaction between these factors is the basis for the availability of the medication administered to the target tissues. Detailed knowledge of the quantitative relationships involved and the changes with age will enable us to make more accurate predictions as to therapeutic, nontherapeutic, and toxic dosages in aging patients.

REFERENCES

Baylis, E. M., Hall, M. S., Lewis, G., and Marks, V.: Effects of renal function on plasma digoxin levels in elderly ambulant patients in domiciliary practice, Br. Med. J. 1:338, 1972.

Castleden, C. M., Kaye, C. M., and Parsons, R. L.: The effect of age on plasma levels of propranolol and practolol in man, Br. J. Clin. Pharmacol. 2:303, 1975.

Davies, D. F., and Shock, N. W.: Age changes in glomerular filtration rate, effective renal plasma flow, and tubular excretory capacity in adult males, J. Clin. Invest. 29:496, 1950.

Ewy, G. A., Kapadia, G. G., Yao, L., Lullin, M., and Marcus, F. I.: Digoxin metabolism in the elderly, Circulation 39:449, 1969.

Feighner, J. P., Robins, E., Guze, S. B., Woodruff, R. A., Jr., Winokur, G., and Munoz, R.: Diagnostic criteria for use in psychiatric research, Arch. Gen. Psychiatry 26:57, 1972.

Friedel, R. O., and Raskind, M. A.: Relationship of Blood Levels of Sinequan to Clinical Effects in the Treatment of Depression in Aged Patients, in Mendels, J. (ed.): *Sinequan, A Monograph of Recent Clinical Studies* (Princeton: Excerpta Medica, 1975), pp. 51–53.

Friedel, R. O., and Raskind, M. A.: Psychopharmacology of Aging, in Elias, M. F., Eleftheriou, B. E., and Elias, P. K. (eds.): *Special Review of Experimental Aging Research: Progress in Biology* (Bar Harbor: E.A.R., 1977).

Garattini, S., Marcucci, F., Morselli, P. L., and Mussini, E.: The Significance of Measuring Blood Levels of Benzodiazepines, in Davies, D. S., and Prichard, B. N. C. (eds.): *Biological Effects of Drugs in Relation to Their Plasma Concentrations* (Baltimore: University Park Press, 1973), pp. 211–25.

Glassman, A. H., Hurwic, M. J., and Perel, J. M.: Plasma binding of imipramine and clinical outcome, Am. J. Psychiatry 130:1367, 1973.

Goldring, W., Chasis, H., Ranges, H. A., and Smith, H. W.: Relations of effective renal blood flow and glomerular filtration to tubular excretory mass in normal man, J. Clin. Invest. 19:739, 1940.

Greenblatt, D. J., and Koch-Weser, J.: Clinical pharmacokinetics, parts 1 and 2, N. Engl. J. Med. 293:702 and 964, 1975.

Greenblatt, D. J., Shader, R. I., and Koch-Weser, J.: Slow absorption of intramuscular chlordiazepoxide, N. Engl. J. Med. 291:1116, 1974.

Gregerman, R. I., and Bierman, E. L.: Aging and hormones, in Williams, R. H. (ed.): *Textbook of Endocrinology* (Philadelphia: W. B. Saunders Co., 1974).

Gregerman, R. I., Gaffney, G. W., and Shock, N. W.: Thyroxine turnover in euthyroid man, with special reference to changes with age, J. Clin. Invest. 41:2065, 1962.

Hillestad, L., Hansen, T., Melsom, H., and Privenes, A.: Diazepam metabolism in normal man: I. Serum concentrations and clinical effects after intravenous, intramuscular, and oral administration, Clin. Pharmacol. Ther. 16: 479, 1974.

Hollister, J. E., Curry, S. H., Derr, J. E., and Kanter, S. L.: Studies of delayed-action medication: V. Plasma levels and urinary excretion of four different dosage forms of chlorpromazine, Clin. Pharmacol. Ther. 11:49, 1970.

Irvine, R. E., Grove, J., Toseland, P. A., and Trounce, J. R.: The effect of age on the hydroxylation of amylobarbitone sodium in man, Br. J. Clin. Pharmacol. 1:41, 1974.

Jenkins, R. G., and Friedel, R. O.: Analysis of tricyclic antidepressants in human plasma by GC/CIMS with selected ion monitoring, J. Pharm. Sci. (in press).

Jori, A., DiSalle, E., and Quadri, A.: Rate of aminopyrine disappearance from plasma in young and aged humans, Pharmacology 8:273, 1972.

Kato, R., and Takanaka, A.: Metabolism of drugs in old rats II. Metabolism *in vivo* and effect of drugs in old rats, Jpn. J. Pharmacol. 18:389, 1968.

Kato, R., Vassanelli, P., Frontino, G., and Chiesera, E.: Variation in the activity of liver microsomal drug metabolizing enzymes in rats in relation to the age, Biochem. Pharmacol. 13:1037, 1964.

Klotz, U., Avant, G. R., Hoyumpa, A., Schenker, S., and Wilkinson, G. R.: The effects of age and liver disease on the disposition and elimination of diazepam in adult man, J. Clin. Invest. 55:347, 1975.

Korenchevsky, V.: *Physiological and Pathological Aging* (New York: Hafner Publishing Co., 1961).

Lasagna, L.: Drug Effects as Modified by Aging, in Moore, J., Merritt, H., and Massilink, R. (eds.): *The Neurologic and Psychiatric Aspects of the Disorders of Aging* (Baltimore: Williams & Wilkins Co., 1956), pp. 83–94.

Leikola, E., and Vartia, K. O.: On penicillin levels in young and geriatric subjects, J. Gerontol. 12:48, 1957.

Mølholm Hansen, J., Kampmann, J., and Laursen, H.: Renal excretion of drugs in the elderly, Lancet 1:1170, 1970.

Oates, J. A., and Shand, D. G.: Are We Measuring the Right Things? The Role of Active Metabolites, in Davies, D. S., and Pritchard, B. N. C. (eds.): *Biological Effects of Drugs in Relation to Their Plasma Concentrations* (Baltimore: University Park Press, 1973), pp. 97–106.

Shader, R. I., Greenblatt, D. J., Harmatz, J. S., Franke, K., and Koch-Weser, J.: Absorption and disposition of chlordiazepoxide in young and elderly male volunteers, J. Clin. Pharmacol. (In press.)

Siersback-Nielsen, K., Mølholm Hansen, J. M., Kampmann, J., and Kristensen, M.: Rapid evaluation of creatinine clearance, Lancet 1:1133, 1971.

Simon, C., Malerczyk, V., Müller, U., and Müller, G.: Zur Pharmacokinetik von Propicillin bei Geriatrischen Patienten im Vergleich zu jungeren Erwachsenen, Dtsch. Med. Wochenschr. 97:1999, 1972.

Thompson, E. N., and Williams, R.: Effects of age on liver function with particular reference to Bromsulphalein excretion, Gut 6:266, 1965.

Vartia, K. O., and Leikola, E.: Serum levels of antibiotics in young and old subjects following administration of dihydrostreptomycin and tetracycline, J. Gerontol. 15:392, 1960.

Watkin, M., and Shock, N. W.: Agewise standard value for C_{In}, C_{PAH}, and Tm_{PAH} in adult males, J. Clin. Invest. 34:969, 1955.

Wilkinson, G. R., and Shand, D. G.: A physiological approach to hepatic drug clearance, Clin. Pharmacol. Ther. 18:377, 1975.

Discussion III

DISCUSSANT: ITZCHAK MARGULEC, M.D., M.P.H.
Medical Director, American Joint Distribution Committee; Associate Director,
Brookdale Institute of Gerontology and Adult Human Development; Visiting
Professor in Social Medicine, Hebrew University-Hadassah Medical School,
Jerusalem, Israel

I'D LIKE to make a few remarks about comprehensive care of the mentally disordered patient.

The approximately 300 million persons 60 years of age and over, in 1970, throughout the world, will double to nearly 600 million by the year 2000, a 100% increase. During this period, the world's population as a whole will increase from 3.6 to 6.5 billion, or about 80%.

For the less developed countries, the proportionate increase of the elder population will be more significant than in the developed countries. The increase in the group aged 60 and above will be about 158%, while the increase in the total population will be about 98%.

How many people, then, will be in the group of the so-called old— 75, 85, and older? And how many mentally disordered people will we have in the world?

In planning geriatric programs, the emphasis should be on all aspects of prevention: medical prevention, environmental prevention; as well as on clinical care and the reintegration of older persons into society.

The holistic approach should be adopted in handling the complex medical needs of the aged, which should always be considered in relation to the family. A system of delivery of geriatric services should include home care, outpatient facilities, and community supports, as well as hospital care for acute and for long-term continuous care. The dynamic approach calls for dealing with elderly persons within the context of their families. To do this at this stage of development, we need, as we say in Israel, those who are *meshuganim l'davar*—"crazy for the cause."

It is good to have enthusiasts, but it is not enough. We need proper staff. We need to train and prepare all the multidisciplined staff needed for care of the aged: health professionals, social workers, occupational therapists, physical therapists, speech therapists, psychologists, volunteer workers.

Medical schools should include in their curriculum the study of adult human development and aging in all its aspects: physiological, psychological, pathological, clinical, epidemiological, and sociological. The possibilities of research in this field should be emphasized in order to challenge new generations of physicians.

Geriatric services should be established as an integral part of the general health services. In developing comprehensive health and social services, we should combine them for adults and the aged. This will be more attractive for the personnel, and they will see this life span from adulthood to advanced age. Services should be available to all the aged who need them, and developed with the close participation of those using the services.

A few words about terminology. We still use the term "custodial care." In 1957 when I was in the United States studying public health, I read with great interest the classical book on chronic diseases by the Commission on Chronic Diseases. They suggested at that time eliminating the term "custodial care." It is a stigma for the patient, for the family, for the care givers. In Israel we have an even worse phrase: "the hopeless patient." I feel that even "nursing care" is not a good term, because it suggests people we have to handle or take care of on a certain level. I hope that we can find a much better term for such care.

While planning needs are urgent, it is essential that we make a serious effort to first understand some of the feelings of the aged, and to define some of their real problems.

One problem is that the aged commonly do not feel useful to the family or to society. There is often a feeling of internal void or boredom. Another problem is the tendency to deny the present to the aged person, forcing him to think of himself as belonging to the past.

The aged individual, like the young, needs to see himself as part of the present: to see the present as important to him, and to see himself as useful in the present.

OPEN DISCUSSION

FROM THE FLOOR: A difficult point for all of us is that there is no exact classification of the neurological entities of the impaired brain in the elderly. In the same patient, one specialist might diagnose cerebral sclerosis, another might call it organic brain syndrome, and still another might say pseudodementia. In addition, there are in the literature such terms as functional dementia, etc. Perhaps it's worth organizing a special discussion about this topic, and elaborating some proposals in order finally to come to a unified classification of these states.

Since I work in the houses for the aged in Israel, I see a large proportion of patients who show confusional states. These seem to be caused by various kinds of memory disorders. Can we clarify the neurological and pathological basis for this impaired memory functioning and make some differentiations?

Are some of the clinical tests better than others in correlating with the various types of pathology?

PROFESSOR ISAACS: Since we don't have specific diagnostic tests that we can apply in life that will tell us the pathology, I think the classification of brain impairment in the elderly should be clinical. We already, of course, have Roth's well-known classification, published many years ago, but perhaps it would need some revision today.

But if we're looking for a clinical classification, why do we look upon the brain as being different from any other organ in the body? We commonly talk about heart failure or liver failure, and I suggest that we talk about brain failure. This is a concept which we have already used for some years, and it was published some years ago by Caird in Glasgow. We talk about brain failure, which allows us to make no etiological presumptions, and leaves the field of pathology and prognosis wide open. We subdivide into acute and chronic brain failure, and we again look in terms of compensated and decompensated brain failure.

These are generally accepted concepts from other fields of disease, and I think they apply very neatly. Within acute brain failure we can further subdivide them. Within chronic brain failure we can make the pathological distinctions. Compensation and decompensation are extremely important, because they enable us to differentiate between the results of pathological tests, on the one hand, which show us the quality or the degree of failure present, and the behavior pattern—so that one can have quite a severe brain failure, which is compensated, and thus presents little management problem. I would suggest that this is a framework on which some generally agreed nosology could very well be arranged.

DOCTOR LIBOW: I agree that we should discuss the classification problem and try to improve on present usage.

There is one subgroup of senile dementia whose initiating event would seem to be diminished cerebral flow. There is another subgroup whose initiating event seems to be based on a primary neuronal tissue decline and secondary decrease of cerebral blood flow.

But still, in many of the papers in the most prestigious journals, these subgroups are combined and we continue to do studies without using existing information.

DOCTOR LEHMANN: Apparently with many dementias, circulation in the brain and vascular activity is comparatively normal, and if the blood flow is diminished, it is often thought to be secondary to diminished metabolic demands of the brain tissue. The primary lesion may be a chemical metabolic lesion of brain tissue—not necessarily a neuronal loss that may be irreversible, but, anyway, a metabolic impairment.

FROM THE FLOOR: I would like to submit that I believe that the nurse is and will be the major care giver for the aged in general, and particularly for the cognitively impaired. This is for a number of reasons. First, because of the nature of nursing, which is supportive, educative, and involved with personal care.

The second reason is that the nurse in most settings, particularly in the community, is the first care giver in primary care. She is the first contact with the patient and with the family.

And thirdly, simply because we are so many everywhere and so much of the time. The nurses are the largest group of suppliers of health care. We are everywhere, and we are there 24 hours a day. So, whether you like it or not, psychiatrists, physicians, and organizers of health services: here we are, take note of us, and please help us fulfill the function that I think we can fulfill so well. Please don't ignore us by believing that there are only physicians and psychiatrists in the world. I don't mean that facetiously. I'm really very sincere in this. It's just that sometimes people forget that other people exist.

Professor Isaacs' model doesn't seem entirely feasible, both because we can't build that fast to supply enough beds, even if it were desirable—and there is also the economic factor. So I think we have to find alternatives, and I believe that the nurse in the community is the answer—whether we call her a public nurse, health visitor, family nurse, community nurse, or whatever.

The nurse is an accepted person, in the family, in the community because she comes in to look after nice things like pregnant women and babies, in addition to the old people. Because she is such an acceptable person, she is there, and she can very often be the first person in early diagnosis, picking up the kinds of things the family and the patient himself are not aware of, because they are so subjective and are used to what is going on. They don't see the subtle changes.

Another role that she has is in the outreach program. I was thinking of the grass-nibbler (mentioned by Doctor Epstein) who doesn't want to come into care, and I don't even know if he should go into care. A nurse could reach out and give him care in a form which is acceptable.

And then third, a major role which the community nurse can fulfill is being a major therapeutic and supportive person to those individuals and families in the home, and I think that Miriam Hirshfeld elaborated on this very nicely.

This brings us to a number of implications. First of all, that of education. If we want nurses to do this, they have to know how to do it. They need knowledge and very specific skills.

Secondly, this kind of care should be integrated into the general family care and then you don't have all the resistance about who is ready to go into caring for the aged.

Further, there is need for supervision and support to the care givers. Regardless of how well they are prepared, they still need support and a chance to ventilate and to share some of the pressures that they're under.

FROM THE FLOOR: I am the medical supervisor for nursing homes of the Ministry of Health in Israel. Most of the big problems that I have every day are connected with the use of drugs in the nursing homes.

We have here heard about the use of drugs for the mentally ill, but the mentally ill are not only mentally ill. They also suffer from other diseases—in the older patient from about six diseases at the same time. That is the problem.

We first treat the mentally ill, and he receives drugs. But on the first day that the patient comes to the nursing home, we find that he is agitated, and he needs something for this. He also needs something for his insomnia. And he brings from home also something for his constipation, because every patient in the nursing home suffers from constipation. He also needs something for pain. He is also anorectic and he is taking some vitamins. So we begin the drug treatment with five different drugs. Then we start the treatment of his mental illness. But he is suffering also from heart disease, and then he is taking something for the blood pressure. He is also taking some diuretic and if he is suffering from angina pains, then also something for this.

But this is not all, because he is also a diabetic, and takes something for that. But that's not all, because he is suffering from a urinary tract infection and he is catheterized and he is taking an antibiotic.

He also suffers from Parkinson's disease and is taking L-dopa and. . . . So at the second day of treatment, the patient is taking more or less 20 different drugs, three or four times a day.

What happens with the interaction of so many different drugs that the patient is taking, and what occurs especially in the old patient with all these drugs? [Applause]

DOCTOR LEHMANN: It's quite characteristic that everybody is amused by all this. It really isn't so amusing. When we get old, we just have all these failures. Nobody thinks it's funny that some people have to wear glasses and false teeth and a hearing aid and use a cane, and a catheter—that's not funny. But when it comes to different medications, all of a sudden—I don't know why—polypharmacy always amuses people.

But somehow all these medications, I think, in this particular case, and for any unfortunate person who has all these problems—they are all indicated and they are all necessary. Older people on occasion just have to be kept together with paper clips and Scotch tape. And these various things are indeed all indicated. Analgesics and hypnotics and circulatory agents and antibiotics and what have you.

There is currently a great deal of study going on focused on the interactions of these drugs. The whole subspecialty of pharmacology is investigating these interactions, and any good physician who is treating a geriatric patient ought to know about such possible interactions. As long as people get old the way they do and fall apart, it's like your car—you have to look at the rust, at the carburetor, at the tires, and so forth. Everything goes to pieces, and you just have to attend to all of it. I'm afraid that can't be helped.

DOCTOR EISDORFER: We run into such problems all the time and must deal with them. There are some solutions however. One is to find out whether the insomnia, the constipation, the pain, and the agitation really require individual drugs or perhaps one drug for depression such as a tricyclic antidepressant. Perhaps we often get ourselves into such difficulties by starting out wrong. A strategy which involves the symptomatic treatment of the aged or any other patients, rather than the nosologic and diagnostic approach or, if you will, the treatment of the underlying condition or disease, could pose serious problems in the long run.

A first step is to decide whether or not we're living in a culture where the aged patient tries to pressure the physician to give him a drug on each visit. This becomes an implicit part of the physician-patient interaction. I say that because I happen to know the data for Israel, which is that the per-patient drug utilization is considerably higher for the same kind of condition than it is in other parts of the world with approximately the same standards for medical care. The physician, the social worker, the nurse—everyone in the health care team—has a responsibility to look at what drugs are used in what ways, and this includes their symbolic as well as pharmacologic properties.

This represents an exciting challenge. The manifestations of drug-drug interactions are becoming a more acute problem throughout the world. With all due respect to Doctor Lehmann, whom I fully support in his statement, even the excellent physician now is running into trouble. We find patients regularly taking 10 to 15 or more drugs, and then borrowing or inheriting others from friends and neighbors, complicated by the pattern in some areas of multiple physicians with limited information. Even a good physician will need some special help with this dilemma.

One partial solution that is emerging in the United States is the strengthening of clinical pharmacology as a subdiscipline of medicine. Clinical pharmacologists spend a good deal of their professional lives evaluating just these drug-drug interactions. We are also witnessing the emergence of experimental programs which involve putting all drug information on computers so that if a physician feels that he or she may be getting into trouble, one can get information. What would be the effect of adding a new ingredient to this stew? If we are talking about a polypharmacologic stew, it's quite important to know about the effects of additions.

MIRIAM HIRSCHFELD: I think that a good nurse could cut down on some of the medication at least. For instance, in insomnia a person's inability to sleep is often caused by anxiety. He wants someone to talk to when he is upset, and might need a backrub, or a cup of warm milk.

You could alleviate constipation, either by the food you give or by exercises. There are several bowel-training methods.

You could definitely cut down on a lot of pain medications, because again they are very often a plea for some attention, for some help. Often these medications are necessary, but often they can be substituted by appropriate nursing intervention.

On vitamin pills, we definitely can cut down by watching a balanced diet. Perhaps not on B_{12}, but on other vitamins, yes. The skilled nurse will be aware of side effects. Let's say, if digoxin is given, it takes a while before side effects and complications are noticed. Diarrhea may be treated with another drug when it is actually a side effect of digoxin.

In Israel where tomatoes and apricots are plentiful, there should be no need to give electrolyte medications as long as an old person is not acutely ill.

On the question of diuretics: if one could manage to plan a diet with less salt and make it palatable with different spices or salt substitutes, as well as encourage the patient's cooperation in keeping the diet, it might be possible to cut down on some of the diuretics.

Antibiotics. If we had, especially in institutions, an environment that could be geared more toward preventing infections—such as changing catheters under antiseptic conditions, or simply keeping a clean (and aseptic) environment—it would be possible to work toward preventing the overuse of antibiotics. Today we seem to consider sterility, aseptic technique, and even handwashing as outdated rituals, since we supposedly have antibiotics to combat infection.

DOCTOR EISDORFER: I think that question has been well answered. It also opens up, I think, the opportunity for an educational program for physicians in collaboration with nurses and other health professionals.

FROM THE FLOOR: Regarding one of the points raised by Doctor Friedel: I am struck by the fact that we need to pay more attention to alteration in so-called circadian or biological rhythms in the elderly. In addition to the other factors mentioned in regard to drug effective absorption, excretion, metabolism, and so forth, biological rhythms clearly play a role in drug effectiveness and patient reaction.

I strongly suspect that these rhythms are quite different among the aged. The little bit we know certainly points in that way. There are really some quite remarkable changes with aging, and certainly sleep patterns are different in elderly people. But we have to start thinking about endocrine changes and endocrine excretion patterns which change biologically and to consider not only those changes we would think of, but also whether they change on a rhythmic basis. There is also quite a variation in how people react to disability—and much that we will have to look at before we fully understand the physiology and thus the care of the older person.

FROM THE FLOOR: This is more of a statement than a question. There are other professionals, staff physicians, and nurses who are also involved with working with the cognitively impaired elderly. The term covers a broader spectrum than the very severely ill patients that have been discussed. We are seeing more and more of the borderline cases coming in, into institutions, into day-care centers, and day hospitals — individuals suffering from memory loss, confusion, and fears which may or not be based on realities. This is a population which might be maintained in the community with proper supportive systems.

The social workers, the occupational therapists, the activity workers are all persons who are concerned with means of working with somewhat impaired persons. We are not directly involved in medication. We do need guidance from physicians, but we are also means of giving information to physicians and nurses on behaviors.

I think there really needs to be more information-sharing among the fields. I think possibly also we need to have another session at which these borderline kinds of individuals are discussed. They don't get handled and medicated in the same fashion that the severely ill do. And in fact, they're much more of a problem.

DOCTOR EISDORFER: The borderline case does represent the larger logistical problem, I believe. One of the things which would have to be considered would be: are we talking about an early intervention in a process of steady decline, or are we talking about two different kinds of people, one of which remains stable at marginal levels? I don't think we have a simple answer.

FROM THE FLOOR: It's an important point, and I think we shouldn't forget it, that institutionalization makes older people become more deteriorated and causes an increase in the mortality rate. In our own area, and especially in the Negev, we work with a lot of people from the Oriental countries, where children and parents live closely, and for them the idea of being sent to homes for the aged is a very strange idea. So we have to encourage the care of the elderly at home. For us the first challenge and the first priority is good home care programs. It's not easy, because most of the elderly patients are treated by general practitioners who are often not aware of geriatrics. We very often see a tendency to treat classical problems, and to neglect the functional aspects of the elderly. We need these physicians to join us.

Epilogue

ISRAEL KATZ, D.S.W.
Director, Brookdale Institute of Gerontology and Adult Human Development,
American Joint Distribution Committee, Givat Ram, Jerusalem, Israel

I HAVE BEEN LISTENING carefully to these presentations and comments. As a student of social policy, I rather acted as a participant-observer of what seemed to me to be enlightening exchanges of biomedical, clinical, and sociomedical contributions to the topic of this workshop. I was asking myself continually, and especially when the term "patient" was used in the context of helping relationships, who is, or should be, my patient? Is it that older mother, her daughter, the network of our health and welfare programs and services, the medical profession, or our society? To me it seemed quite obvious that if our efforts are to be effective, the question "Who is my patient?" becomes a very crucial one. The patient is certainly not he alone who has conventionally been perceived and conceived as the receiver of aid and assistance. The entire society must be sensitized to the needs of and to the value of the aged.

Some time ago, a very prestigious research organization made the point that in case of atomic disaster, people who were 55 years or over should not be cared for. Caring for them, while assuming some kind of survival of mankind, would not make sense! And yet, our group here addressed itself to this very group of people and to its increasing number in our societies in the future.

Indeed, the population of older citizens will increase, but older people have been and will remain a marginal group in all our countries. As a marginal group the aged have many social characteristics of marginality and yet they are also different from certain other marginal groups.

The poor, for example, another marginal group, may be worse off today in many ways than they were in some of our countries in the 1920s or the 1930s. At that time more people were poor than today.

161

As the middle classes have increased in all our welfare states, the poor have become a proportionately smaller group and thus a rather weaker agent of change.

Viewing the aged as a growing group, marginal though it remains, may reinforce one's optimism as to the opportunities to bring about change for the improvement of its welfare. However, the concept of welfare is, and will be, changing too, and the demands of peoples' welfare on scarce resources are increasing enormously. It appears that the concept of welfare has broadened and continues to expand so that it now includes everything that people would rather have than be without. Health; human and social welfare; a high standard of living; capital; property; amount and use of leisure; the environment in which people work, live, and retire into; status; prestige, and meaningful social roles are only some of the rather general areas, the existence and expansion of which depend on the distribution of material and nonmaterial resources. Such distributions are determined by political processes and decisions in all our countries. It is not at all clear whether or not the aged will fare better, relative to other groups, in the future than they have in the past. Be that as it may, it seems to me that only by more deliberate, aggressive, and concerted interventions of a multidimensional nature will it be possible to advance the health and welfare of older people. To do so, broader scientific, professional, and political coalitions will be required. Doctors, psychologists, sociologists, political scientists, economists, social workers, nurses, administrators, politicians, and many other experts and citizens in our communities must, therefore, be encouraged to increasingly raise and face the question of "Who is my patient?"

We do hope that the Brookdale Institute of Gerontology and Human Development of the American Joint Distribution Committee in Jerusalem will join with you and contribute to a sharper definition of the targets to be attacked for the progress of health and welfare of individuals, families, and communities in our countries.

Index

Hypochondriacal person: and stress, 107
Hypoglycemia: causing acute mental changes, 84
Hyponatremia: causing acute mental changes, 84–85
Hypothyroidism: causing acute mental changes, 84

I

Illness: physical, and testing difficulties, 23
Imipramine: for depression, 133–134
Indomethacin: causing psychotic behavior, 83
Information and referral, 97–104
  discussion of, 105–106
  functions of, 98–99
  services
    as part of comprehensive care, 100–101
    definitions of, 98
    development of, 98
    operational model, 101–102
    telephone, 102–103
Information test (see Memory and Information Test)
Insomnia: drugs for, 131–132
Integrity (see Nursing care, conservation of integrity)
Intelligence
  assessment, difficulties in, 21–22
  blood pressure and, 37–38
  EEG and, 37
  test
    scores, 63–65
    standardized, 16
Irritability: drugs for, 132–133
Isotope cisternography, 76, 77

K

Ketoacidotic state: and acute mental change, 84

L

Laboratory tests: for investigation of senile dementia, 76–77

Lactic acidosis syndrome: and acute mental changes, 84
Largactil: for insomnia, 132
Learning: and psychological evaluation, 65–66
Lethargy: drugs for, 135
Librium (see Chlordiazepoxide)
Life event changes, and stress, 32–35
  life span analysis of, 35–36
Liver conditions: and mental changes, 86
Lung conditions: and mental changes, 86

M

MAO inhibitors, 133
Medical practitioner, 89–95
Medications (see Drugs)
Mellaril: for insomnia, 132
Memory
  and Information Test (see below)
  psychological evaluation and, 65–66
  rating scale, 17–18
Memory and Information Test
  example of, 17
  Newcastle upon Tyne study, 19–20
  shortened form of, 24
Mental
  changes, potentially reversible, causes of
    acute, 81–86
    chronic, 86–87
  disease, chronic, relations between chronic brain syndrome and, 48–52
  status evaluation technique, FROMAJE, 77–81
  testing, discussion of, 49
Meprobamate: for daytime sedation, 133
Metabolic imbalance: causing acute mental changes, 83–85
Methylphenidate: for lethargy, 135
Metrazol: for lethargy, 135
Microtubules, 6
Mini-Mult, 66